Teen Health Series

Allergy Information For Teens, Third Edition

Allergy Information For Teens, Third Edition

Health Tips About Allergic Reactions To Food, Pollen, Mold, And Other Substances

Including Facts About Diagnosing, Treating, And Preventing Allergic Responses And Complications

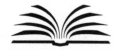

OMNIGRAPHICS
615 Griswold, Ste. 901
Detroit, MI 48226

Bibliographic Note
Because this page cannot legibly accommodate all the copyright notices, the Bibliographic Note portion of the Preface constitutes an extension of the copyright notice.

* * *

OMNIGRAPHICS
Siva Ganesh Maharaja, *Managing Editor*

* * *

Copyright © 2018 Omnigraphics

ISBN 978-0-7808-1593-3
E-ISBN 978-0-7808-1594-0

Library of Congress Cataloging-in-Publication Data

Names: Omnigraphics, Inc., issuing body.

Title: Allergy information for teens: health tips about allergic reactions to food, pollen, mold, and other substances including facts about diagnosing, treating, and preventing allergic responses and complications.

Description: Third edition. | Detroit, MI: Omnigraphics, Inc., [2018] | Series: Teen health series | Audience: Grade 9 to 12. | Includes bibliographical references and index.

Identifiers: LCCN 2017044871 (print) | LCCN 2017045901 (ebook) | ISBN 9780780815940 (eBook) | ISBN 9780780815933 (hardcover: alk. paper)

Subjects: LCSH: Allergy. | Allergy in children. | Food allergy. | Insect allergy.

Classification: LCC RC584 (ebook) | LCC RC584.A45 2018 (print) | DDC 616.9700835--dc23

LC record available at https://lccn.loc.gov/2017044871

Table Of Contents

Preface

Part One: Allergy Overview

Chapter 1——Allergies: The Basic Facts 3

Chapter 2——The Immune System And Its Role In
Allergies 7

Chapter 3——The Respiratory System And How It Works 17

Chapter 4——Cold, Flu, Or Allergy? 23

Chapter 5——When You Should See An Allergist 27

Chapter 6——Lung Function Tests For Breathing
Problems 31

Chapter 7——Patch Tests For Allergies 37

Chapter 8——Allergy Blood Test 41

Chapter 9——Allergy Shots (Immunotherapy) 45

Chapter 10—Medications Used To Treat Allergic
Symptoms 53

Chapter 11—Epinephrine Injections For
Life-Threatening Allergic Reactions 57

Part Two: Allergy Symptoms And Complications

Chapter 12—Coughing And Sneezing 63

Chapter 13—Allergic Rhinitis 71

Chapter 14—Sinusitis 77

Chapter 15—Asthma And Allergies 81

Chapter 16—Hypersensitivity Pneumonitis 85

Chapter 17—Eye Allergies 97

Chapter 18—Contact Dermatitis And Latex Allergy 103

Chapter 19—Atopic Dermatitis (Eczema) 109

Chapter 20—Urticaria (Hives).. 115

Chapter 21—Anaphylaxis And Exercise-Induced
Anaphylaxis 119

Chapter 22—Climate Change And Respiratory
Allergies 123

Part Three: Food Allergies And Intolerances

Chapter 23—Food Allergies: What You Need To Know 127

Chapter 24—Food Allergy And Related Disorders 133

Chapter 25—Peanut And Tree Nut Allergies.................................... 137

Chapter 26—Wheat Allergy 143

Chapter 27—Soy Allergy 145

Chapter 28—Dark Chocolate And Milk Allergies 149

Chapter 29—Seafood Allergy.. 155

Chapter 30—Lactose Intolerance 159

Chapter 31—Egg Allergy 167

Chapter 32—Gluten Intolerance (Celiac Disease)........................... 171

Chapter 33—Scombrotoxin (Histamine) Poisoning........................ 183

Chapter 34—Sulfite Sensitivity 187

Part Four: Other Common Allergy Triggers

Chapter 35—Pollen Allergies... 195

Chapter 36—Pet Allergies.. 199

Chapter 37—Allergies And Other Health
Effects Of Mold... 203

Chapter 38—Cockroach Allergy... 209

Chapter 39—Dust Mites 213

Chapter 40—Smoking 217

Chapter 41—Sting Allergies 221

Chapter 42—Nickel Allergy 227

Chapter 43—Hair Dye Allergy 235

Chapter 44—Fragrance Allergy 241

Chapter 45—Lanolin Allergy 245

Chapter 46—Formaldehyde Allergy 249

Part Five: Managing Allergies In Daily Life

Chapter 47—When Breathing Becomes Bothersome 255

Chapter 48—How To Control Seasonal Allergies 259

Chapter 49—Managing Indoor Air Quality 263

Chapter 50—Asthma Management At School 269

Chapter 51—Using Cosmetics Safely 273

Chapter 52—Use Caution With Face Painting And
Tattoos 277

Chapter 53—Nail Care Product Safety 283

Chapter 54—Skin Care Concerns For People With
Eczema 287

Chapter 55—Have Food Allergies? Read The Label 293

Chapter 56—The Food Allergen Labeling and
Consumer Protection Act (FALCPA) 299

Chapter 57—Going Out To Eat With Food Allergies 305

Chapter 58—Food Allergy Lab Fits On Your Keychain 309

Chapter 59—Working With A Dietitian 313

Chapter 60—A Food Diary Can Reduce Risk Of
             Reactions.. 317

Chapter 61—Egg Allergies And Vaccines.. 319

Part Six: If You Need More Information

Chapter 62—Resources For Allergy Information............................... 325

Chapter 63—Finding Recipes Online If You Have
             Food Allergies.. 337

Index 343

Preface

About This Book

According to the Centers for Disease Control and Prevention's (CDC) National Center for Health Statistics, just under 6% of people under 18 have food allergies. Other common allergies for people under the age of 18 include respiratory and skin allergies.

The consequences of allergic diseases vary considerably. For some people, the symptoms are merely a transient annoyance—occasional sniffles, sneezes, or mild itching. Others endure persistent, more severe symptoms that can disrupt education and relationships, hamper the adoption of healthy lifestyle choices, and hinder overall well-being. Chronic symptoms can lead to additional health concerns, such as the development of asthma. In some people with severe allergies, the consequences can even be deadly.

Allergy Information For Teens, Third Edition provides updated information about a wide variety of allergic reactions, including common symptoms, diagnostic tools, and prevention strategies. It recounts what is currently known about the causes of allergies and the role the immune system plays in their development. It presents facts about rhinitis, sinusitis, dermatitis, urticaria (hives), anaphylaxis, and other types of symptoms produced by encounters with allergens. It also looks at the substances responsible for triggering these types of symptoms, including specific foods, animals, pollens, and chemicals. A special section on managing allergies in daily life outlines ways to avoid allergy triggers, handle medication at school, and cope with other challenges. The book concludes with resource directories for learning more about allergies and finding recipes to aid in the management of food allergies.

How To Use This Book

This book is divided into parts and chapters. Parts focus on broad areas of interest; chapters are devoted to single topics within a part.

Part One: Allergy Overview explains the biological processes that lead to the development of allergies and how allergy symptoms are detected and differentiated from symptoms due to other causes. It also provides facts about some of the most commonly used allergy treatments and the use of epinephrine injections for life-threatening allergic reactions.

Part Two: Allergy Symptoms And Complications provides details about various ways allergic reactions can be identified and how they impact health. It discusses signs that may indicate breathing complications, and it explains how allergies can lead to the development of chronic respiratory illnesses. Other allergic symptoms, including those that affect the eyes and skin, are also discussed, and the part concludes with a chapter on how climate changes can affect allergies.

Part Three: Food Allergies And Intolerances describes the differences between allergies and other adverse biological reactions to ingested substances. Individual chapters address the foods that are most commonly involved in allergic reactions, including nuts, grains, milk, chocolate, eggs, and seafood. The most common intolerances and sensitivities—those to lactose, gluten, histamine, and sulfites—are also addressed.

Part Four: Other Common Allergy Triggers discusses some of the most frequently encountered substances in the indoor and outdoor environments that elicit allergic responses. These include allergies to pollens, pet dander, mold, and dust mites. Allergies to specific chemicals, including latex, nickel, and those that are frequently used in cosmetics, toiletries, clothing, and household products are also explained.

Part Five: Managing Allergies In Daily Life provides tips for people with allergies about minimizing the exacerbation of symptoms and maintaining an optimal quality of life. It discusses allergy-related medications in schools, offers suggestions for the safe use of cosmetics and skin care products, and provides additional suggestions for people with food allergies.

Part Six: If You Need More Information includes a directory of organizations to provide further information about allergies and a list of online resources and mobile applications for allergen-free recipes.

Bibliographic Note

This volume contains documents and excerpts from publications issued by the following government agencies: Agency for Healthcare Research and Quality (AHRQ); Agency for Toxic Substances and Disease Registry (ATSDR); Centers for Disease Control and Prevention (CDC); Genetic and Rare Diseases Information Center (GARD); LiverTox®; National Center for Biotechnology Information (NCBI); National Center for Complementary and Alternative Medicine (NCCAM); National Heart, Lung, and Blood Institute (NHLBI); National Institute of Allergy and Infectious Diseases (NIAID); National

Institute of Arthritis and Musculoskeletal and Skin Diseases (NIAMS); National Institute of Biomedical Imaging and Bioengineering (NIBIB); National Institute of Diabetes and Digestive and Kidney Diseases (NIDDK); National Institute of Environmental Health Sciences (NIEHS); National Institutes of Health (NIH); *NIH News in Health*; Office of Disease Prevention and Health Promotion (ODPHP); U.S. Department of Agriculture (USDA); U.S. Environmental Protection Agency (EPA); and U.S. Food and Drug Administration (FDA).

It may also contain original material produced by Omnigraphics and reviewed by medical consultants.

The photograph on the front cover is © Michael Moloney.

Medical Review

Omnigraphics contracts with a team of qualified, senior medical professionals who serve as medical consultants for the *Teen Health Series*. As necessary, medical consultants review reprinted and originally written material for currency and accuracy. Citations including the phrase, Reviewed (month, year)" indicate material reviewed by this team. Medical consultation services are provided to the *Teen Health Series* editors by:

Dr. Vijayalakshmi, MBBS, DGO, MD
Dr. Senthil Selvan, MBBS, DCH, MD
Dr. K. Sivanandham, MBBS, DCH, MS (Research), PhD

About The *Teen Health Series*

At the request of librarians serving today's young adults, the *Teen Health Series* was developed as a specially focused set of volumes within Omnigraphics' *Health Reference Series*. Each volume deals comprehensively with a topic selected according to the needs and interests of people in middle school and high school. Teens seeking preventive guidance, information about disease warning signs, medical statistics, and risk factors for health problems will find answers to their questions in the *Teen Health Series*. The *Series*, however, is not intended to serve as a tool for diagnosing illness, in prescribing treatments, or as a substitute for the physician/patient relationship. All people concerned about medical symptoms or the possibility of disease are encouraged to seek professional care from an appropriate healthcare provider.

If there is a topic you would like to see addressed in a future volume of the *Teen Health Series*, please write to:

Editor
Teen Health Series
Omnigraphics
615 Griswold, Ste. 901
Detroit, MI 48226

A Note About Spelling And Style

Teen Health Series editors use *Stedman's Medical Dictionary* as an authority for questions related to the spelling of medical terms and the *Chicago Manual of Style* for questions related to grammatical structures, punctuation, and other editorial concerns. Consistent adherence is not always possible, however, because the individual volumes within the *Series* include many documents from a wide variety of different producers and copyright holders, and the editor's primary goal is to present material from each source as accurately as is possible following the terms specified by each document's producer. This sometimes means that information in different chapters may follow other guidelines and alternate spelling authorities. For example, occasionally a copyright holder may require that eponymous terms be shown in possessive forms (Crohn's disease vs. Crohn disease) or that British spelling norms be retained (leukaemia vs. leukemia).

Part One
Allergy Overview

Chapter 1

Allergies: The Basic Facts

What Is Allergy?

An allergy is a reaction by your immune system to something that does not bother most other people. People who have allergies often are sensitive to more than one thing. Substances that often cause reactions are:

- Pollen

- Dust mites

- Mold spores

- Pet dander

- Food

- Insect stings

- Medicines

Normally, your immune system fights germs. It is your body's defense system. In most allergic reactions, however, it is responding to a false alarm. Genes and the environment probably both play a role.

Allergies can cause a variety of symptoms such as a runny nose, sneezing, itching, rashes, swelling, or asthma. Allergies can range from minor to severe. Anaphylaxis is a severe

About This Chapter: Text under the heading "What Is Allergy?" is excerpted from "Allergy," MedlinePlus, National Institutes of Health (NIH), July 6, 2015; Text beginning with the heading "What's The Problem?" is excerpted from "Allergies," Center for Disease Control and Prevention (CDC), September 15, 2017.

reaction that can be life-threatening. Doctors use skin and blood tests to diagnose allergies. Treatments include medicines, allergy shots, and avoiding the substances that cause the reactions.

What's The Problem?

Allergies are the 6th leading cause of chronic illness in the United States with an annual cost in excess of $18 billion. More than 50 million Americans suffer from allergies each year. Allergies are an overreaction of the immune system to substances that generally do not affect other individuals. These substances, or allergens, can cause sneezing, coughing, and itching. Allergic reactions range from merely bothersome to life-threatening. Some allergies are seasonal, like hay fever. Allergies have also been associated with chronic conditions like sinusitis and asthma.

Who's At Risk?

Anyone may have or develop an allergy—from a baby born with an allergy to cow's milk, to a child who gets poison ivy, to a senior citizen who develops hives after taking a new medication.

Can It Be Prevented?

Allergies can generally not be prevented but allergic reactions can be. Once a person knows they are allergic to a certain substance, they can avoid contact with the allergen. Strategies for doing this include being in an air conditioned environment during peak hay fever season, avoiding certain foods, and eliminating dust mites and animal dander from the home. They can also control the allergy by reducing or eliminating the symptoms. Strategies include taking medication to counteract reactions or minimize symptoms and being immunized with allergy injection therapy.

> Medications containing antihistamines, drugs which counteract the effect of histamines, can help relieve many different types of allergies, including hay fever and food allergies. But some antihistamines can make you feel drowsy, unfocused, and slow to react. If not taken responsibly and according to directions, they can pose a danger to your health and safety.
>
> *(Source: "Allergy Meds Could Affect Your Driving," U.S. Food and Drug Administration (FDA).)*

The Bottom Line

- The most common allergic diseases include:

  - Hay fever

  - Asthma

  - Conjunctivitis

  - Hives

  - Eczema

  - Dermatitis

  - Sinusitis

- Food allergies are most prevalent in young children and are frequently outgrown.

- Latex allergies are a reaction to the proteins in latex rubber, a substance used in gloves, condoms, and other products.

- Bees, hornets, wasps, yellow jackets, and fire ants can cause insect sting allergies.

- Allergies to drugs, like penicillin, can affect any tissue or organ in the body.

Anaphylaxis is the most severe allergic reaction. Symptoms include flush; tingling of the palms of the hands, soles of the feet or lips; light headedness, and chest tightness. If not treated, these can progress into seizures, cardiac arrhythmia, shock, and respiratory distress. Anaphylaxis can result in death. Food, latex, insect sting, and drug allergies can all result in anaphylaxis.

Food Allergy Among U.S. Children: Trends In Prevalence And Hospitalizations

- In 2007, approximately 3 million children under age 18 years (3.9%) were reported to have a food or digestive allergy in the previous 12 months.

- From 1997 to 2007, the prevalence of reported food allergy increased 18 percent among children under age 18 years.

- Children with food allergy are two to four times more likely to have other related conditions such as asthma and other allergies, compared with children without food allergies.

- From 2004 to 2006, there were approximately 9,500 hospital discharges per year with a diagnosis related to food allergy among children under age 18 years.

(Source: "Food Allergy Among U.S. Children: Trends In Prevalence And Hospitalizations," Centers for Disease Control and Prevention (CDC).)

Chapter 2

The Immune System And Its Role In Allergies

What Is The Immune System?

The immune system is a network of cells, tissues, and organs that work together to defend the body against attacks by "foreign" invaders. These are primarily microbes—tiny organisms such as bacteria, parasites, and fungi that can cause infections. Viruses also cause infections, but are too primitive to be classified as living organisms. The human body provides an ideal environment for many microbes. It is the immune system's job to keep them out or, failing that, to seek out and destroy them.

When the immune system hits the wrong target, however, it can unleash a torrent of disorders, including allergic diseases, arthritis, and a form of diabetes. If the immune system is crippled, other kinds of diseases result.

The immune system is amazingly complex. It can recognize and remember millions of different enemies, and it can produce secretions (release of fluids) and cells to match up with and wipe out nearly all of them.

The secret to its success is an elaborate and dynamic communications network. Millions and millions of cells, organized into sets and subsets, gather like clouds of bees swarming around a hive and pass information back and forth in response to an infection. Once immune cells receive the alarm, they become activated and begin to produce powerful chemicals. These substances allow the cells to regulate their own growth and behavior, enlist other immune cells, and direct the new recruits to trouble spots.

About This Chapter: Text under the heading "What Is The Immune System?" is excerpted from "What Is The Immune System?" Vaccines.gov, U.S. Department of Health and Human Services (HHS), January 2017; Text beginning with the heading "Function Of The Immune System" is excerpted from "Immune System Research," National Institute of Allergy and Infectious Diseases (NIAID), July 11, 2016.

Although scientists have learned much about the immune system, they continue to study how the body launches attacks that destroy invading microbes, infected cells, and tumors while ignoring healthy tissues. New technologies for identifying individual immune cells are now allowing scientists to determine quickly which targets are triggering an immune response. Improvements in microscopy are permitting the first-ever observations of living B cells, T cells, and other cells as they interact within lymph nodes and other body tissues.

In addition, scientists are rapidly unraveling the genetic blueprints that direct the human immune response, as well as those that dictate the biology of bacteria, viruses, and parasites. The combination of new technology and expanded genetic information will no doubt reveal even more about how the body protects itself from disease.

Function Of The Immune System

The overall function of the immune system is to prevent or limit infection. An example of this principle is found in immune-compromised people, including those with genetic immune disorders, immune debilitating infections like human immunodeficiency virus (HIV), and even pregnant women, who are susceptible to a range of microbes that typically do not cause infection in healthy individuals.

The immune system can distinguish between normal, healthy cells, and unhealthy cells by recognizing a variety of "danger" cues called danger associated molecular patterns (DAMPs). Cells may be unhealthy because of infection or because of cellular damage caused by noninfectious agents like sunburn or cancer. Infectious microbes such as viruses and bacteria release another set of signals recognized by the immune system called pathogen associated molecular patterns (PAMPs).

When the immune system first recognizes these signals, it responds to address the problem. If an immune response cannot be activated when there is sufficient need, problems arise, like infection. On the other hand, when an immune response is activated without a real threat or is not turned off once the danger passes, different problems arise, such as allergic reactions and autoimmune disease.

The immune system is complex and pervasive. There are numerous cell types that either circulate throughout the body or reside in a particular tissue. Each cell type plays a unique role, with different ways of recognizing problems, communicating with other cells, and performing their functions. By understanding all the details behind this network, researchers may optimize immune responses to confront specific issues, ranging from infections to cancer.

Location Of The Cells

All immune cells come from precursors in the bone marrow and develop into mature cells through a series of changes that can occur in different parts of the body.

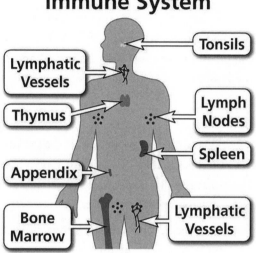

Figure 2.1. Immune System

(Source: "Immune System," AIDSinfo, U.S. Department of Health and Human Services (HHS).)

Skin: The skin is usually the first line of defense against microbes. Skin cells produce and secrete important antimicrobial proteins, and immune cells can be found in specific layers of skin.

Bone marrow: The bone marrow contains stems cells that can develop into a variety of cell types. The common myeloid progenitor stem cell in the bone marrow is the precursor to innate immune cells—neutrophils, eosinophils, basophils, mast cells, monocytes, dendritic cells, and macrophages—that are important first line responders to infection.

The common lymphoid progenitor stem cell leads to adaptive immune cells—B cells and T cells—that are responsible for mounting responses to specific microbes based on previous encounters (immunological memory). Natural killer (NK) cells also are derived from the common lymphoid progenitor and share features of both innate and adaptive immune cells, as they provide immediate defenses like innate cells but also may be retained as memory cells like adaptive cells. B, T, and NK cells also are called lymphocytes.

Bloodstream: Immune cells constantly circulate throughout the bloodstream, patrolling for problems. When blood tests are used to monitor white blood cells, another term for immune cells, a snapshot of the immune system is taken. If a cell type is either scarce or overabundant in the bloodstream, this may reflect a problem.

Thymus: T cells mature in the thymus, a small organ located in the upper chest.

Lymphatic system: The lymphatic system is a network of vessels and tissues composed of lymph, an extracellular fluid, and lymphoid organs, such as lymph nodes. The lymphatic system is a conduit for travel and communication between tissues and the bloodstream. Immune cells are carried through the lymphatic system and converge in lymph nodes, which are found throughout the body.

Lymph nodes are a communication hub where immune cells sample information brought in from the body. For instance, if adaptive immune cells in the lymph node recognize pieces of a microbe brought in from a distant area, they will activate, replicate, and leave the lymph node to circulate and address the pathogen. Thus, doctors may check patients for swollen lymph nodes, which may indicate an active immune response.

Spleen: The spleen is an organ located behind the stomach. While it is not directly connected to the lymphatic system, it is important for processing information from the bloodstream. Immune cells are enriched in specific areas of the spleen, and upon recognizing bloodborne pathogens, they will activate and respond accordingly.

Mucosal tissue: Mucosal surfaces are prime entry points for pathogens, and specialized immune hubs are strategically located in mucosal tissues like the respiratory tract and gut. For instance, Peyer's patches are important areas in the small intestine where immune cells can access samples from the gastrointestinal tract.

Features Of An Immune Response

An immune response is generally divided into innate and adaptive immunity. Innate immunity occurs immediately, when circulating innate cells recognize a problem. Adaptive immunity occurs later, as it relies on the coordination and expansion of specific adaptive immune cells. Immune memory follows the adaptive response, when mature adaptive cells, highly specific to the original pathogen, are retained for later use.

Innate Immunity

Innate immune cells express genetically encoded receptors, called Toll-like receptors (TLRs), which recognize general danger- or pathogen-associated patterns. Collectively, these receptors can broadly recognize viruses, bacteria, fungi, and even noninfectious problems. However, they cannot distinguish between specific strains of bacteria or viruses.

There are numerous types of innate immune cells with specialized functions. They include neutrophils, eosinophils, basophils, mast cells, monocytes, dendritic cells, and macrophages. Their main feature is the ability to respond quickly and broadly when a problem arises, typically leading to inflammation. Innate immune cells also are important for activating adaptive immunity. Innate cells are critical for host defense, and disorders in innate cell function may cause chronic susceptibility to infection.

Adaptive Immunity

Adaptive immune cells are more specialized, with each adaptive B or T cell bearing unique receptors, B-cell receptors (BCRs) and T-cell receptors (TCRs), that recognize specific signals rather than general patterns. Each receptor recognizes an antigen, which is simply any molecule that may bind to a BCR or TCR. Antigens are derived from a variety of sources including pathogens, host cells, and allergens. Antigens are typically processed by innate immune cells and presented to adaptive cells in the lymph nodes.

The genes for BCRs and TCRs are randomly rearranged at specific cell maturation stages, resulting in unique receptors that may potentially recognize anything. Random generation of receptors allows the immune system to respond to new or unforeseen problems. This concept is especially important because environments may frequently change, for instance when seasons change or a person relocates, and pathogens are constantly evolving to survive. Because BCRs and TCRs are so specific, adaptive cells may only recognize one strain of a particular pathogen, unlike innate cells, which recognize broad classes of pathogens. In fact, a group of adaptive cells that recognize the same strain will likely recognize different areas of that pathogen.

If a B or T cell has a receptor that recognizes an antigen from a pathogen and also receives cues from innate cells that something is wrong, the B or T cell will activate, divide, and disperse to address the problem. B cells make antibodies, which neutralize pathogens, rendering them harmless. T cells carry out multiple functions, including killing infected cells and activating or recruiting other immune cells. The adaptive response has a system of checks and balances to prevent unnecessary activation that could cause damage to the host. If a B or T cell is autoreactive, meaning its receptor recognizes antigens from the body's own cells, the cell will be deleted. Also, if a B or T cell does not receive signals from innate cells, it will not be optimally activated.

Immune memory is a feature of the adaptive immune response. After B or T cells are activated, they expand rapidly. As the problem resolves, cells stop dividing and are retained in the body as memory cells. The next time this same pathogen enters the body, a memory cell is already poised to react and can clear away the pathogen before it establishes itself.

Vaccination

Vaccination, or immunization, is a way to train your immune system against a specific pathogen. Vaccination achieves immune memory without an actual infection, so the body is prepared when the virus or bacterium enters. Saving time is important to prevent a pathogen from establishing itself and infecting more cells in the body.

An effective vaccine will optimally activate both the innate and adaptive response. An immunogen is used to activate the adaptive immune response so that specific memory cells are generated. Because BCRs and TCRs are unique, some memory cells are simply better at eliminating the pathogen. The goal of vaccine design is to select immunogens that will generate the most effective and efficient memory response against a particular pathogen. Adjuvants, which are important for activating innate immunity, can be added to vaccines to optimize the immune response. Innate immunity recognizes broad patterns, and without innate responses, adaptive immunity cannot be optimally achieved.

Immune Tolerance

Tolerance is the prevention of an immune response against a particular antigen. For instance, the immune system is generally tolerant of self-antigens, so it does not usually attack the body's own cells, tissues, and organs. However, when tolerance is lost, disorders like autoimmune disease or food allergy may occur. Tolerance is maintained in a number of ways:

- When adaptive immune cells mature, there are several checkpoints in place to eliminate autoreactive cells. If a B cell produces antibodies that strongly recognize host cells, or if a T cell strongly recognizes self-antigen, they are deleted.

- Nevertheless, there are autoreactive immune cells present in healthy individuals. Autoreactive immune cells are kept in a nonreactive, or anergic, state. Even though they recognize the body's own cells, they do not have the ability to react and cannot cause host damage.

- Regulatory immune cells circulate throughout the body to maintain tolerance. Besides limiting autoreactive cells, regulatory cells are important for turning an immune response off after the problem is resolved. They can act as drains, depleting areas of essential nutrients that surrounding immune cells need for activation or survival.

- Some locations in the body are called immunologically privileged sites. These areas, like the eye and brain, do not typically elicit strong immune responses. Part of this is because of physical barriers, like the blood-brain barrier, that limit the degree to which immune cells may enter. These areas also may express higher levels of suppressive cytokines to prevent a robust immune response.

Fetomaternal tolerance is the prevention of a maternal immune response against a developing fetus. Major histocompatibility complex (MHC) proteins help the immune system distinguish between host and foreign cells. MHC also is called human leukocyte antigen (HLA). By expressing paternal MHC or HLA proteins and paternal antigens, a fetus can potentially trigger the mother's immune system. However, there are several barriers that may prevent this from occurring: The placenta reduces the exposure of the fetus to maternal immune cells, the proteins expressed on the outer layer of the placenta may limit immune recognition, and regulatory cells and suppressive signals may play a role.

Transplantation of a donor tissue or organ requires appropriate MHC or HLA matching to limit the risk of rejection. Because MHC or HLA matching is rarely complete, transplant recipients must continuously take immunosuppressive drugs, which can cause complications like higher susceptibility to infection and some cancers. Researchers are developing more targeted ways to induce tolerance to transplanted tissues and organs while leaving protective immune responses intact.

Disorders Of The Immune System

Complications arise when the immune system does not function properly. Some issues are less pervasive, such as pollen allergy, while others are extensive, such as genetic disorders that wipe out the presence or function of an entire set of immune cells.

Immune Deficiencies

Immune deficiencies may be temporary or permanent. Temporary immune deficiency can be caused by a variety of sources that weaken the immune system. Common infections, including influenza and mononucleosis, can suppress the immune system.

When immune cells are the target of infection, severe immune suppression can occur. For example, HIV specifically infects T cells, and their elimination allows for secondary infections by other pathogens. Patients receiving chemotherapy, bone marrow transplants, or immuno-suppressive drugs experience weakened immune systems until immune cell levels are restored. Pregnancy also suppresses the maternal immune system, increasing susceptibility to infections by common microbes.

Primary immune deficiency diseases (PIDDs) are inherited genetic disorders and tend to cause chronic susceptibility to infection. There are over 150 PIDDs, and almost all are considered rare (affecting fewer than 200,000 people in the United States). They may result from altered immune signaling molecules or the complete absence of mature immune cells. For instance, X-linked severe combined immunodeficiency (SCID) is caused by a mutation in a signaling receptor gene, rendering immune cells insensitive to multiple cytokines. Without the growth and activation signals delivered by cytokines, immune cell subsets, particularly T and natural killer cells, fail to develop normally. The National Institute of Allergy and Infectious Diseases (NIAID) Primary Immune Deficiency Clinic was established with the goal of accepting all PIDD patients for examination to provide a disease diagnosis and better treatment recommendations.

Allergy

Allergies are a form of hypersensitivity reaction, typically in response to harmless environmental allergens like pollen or food. Hypersensitivity reactions are divided into four classes. Class I, II, and III are caused by antibodies, IgE or IgG, which are produced by B cells in response to an allergen. Overproduction of these antibodies activates immune cells like basophils and mast cells, which respond by releasing inflammatory chemicals like histamine. Class IV reactions are caused by T cells, which may either directly cause damage themselves or activate macrophages and eosinophils that damage host cells.

Autoimmune Diseases

Autoimmune diseases occur when self-tolerance is broken. Self-tolerance breaks when adaptive immune cells that recognize host cells persist unchecked. B cells may produce antibodies targeting host cells, and active T cells may recognize self-antigen. This amplifies when they recruit and activate other immune cells.

Autoimmunity is either organ-specific or systemic, meaning it affects the whole body. For instance, type I diabetes is organ-specific and caused by immune cells erroneously recognizing insulin-producing pancreatic β cells as foreign. However, systemic lupus erythematosus, commonly called lupus, can result from antibodies that recognize antigens expressed by nearly all healthy cells. Autoimmune diseases have a strong genetic component, and with advances in gene sequencing tools, researchers have a better understanding of what may contribute to specific diseases.

Sepsis

Sepsis may refer to an infection of the bloodstream, or it can refer to a systemic inflammatory state caused by the uncontrolled, broad release of cytokines that quickly activate immune cells throughout the body. Sepsis is an extremely serious condition and is typically triggered by an infection. However, the damage itself is caused by cytokines (the adverse response is sometimes referred to as a "cytokine storm.") The systemic release of cytokines may lead to loss of blood pressure, resulting in septic shock and possible multi-organ failure.

Cancer

Some forms of cancer are directly caused by the uncontrolled growth of immune cells. Leukemia is cancer caused by white blood cells, which is another term for immune cells. Lymphoma is cancer caused by lymphocytes, which is another term for adaptive B or T cells. Myeloma is cancer caused by plasma cells, which are mature B cells. Unrestricted growth of any of these cell types causes cancer.

In addition, an emerging concept is that cancer progression may partially result from the ability of cancer cells to avoid immune detection. The immune system is capable of removing infectious pathogens and dangerous host cells like tumors. Cancer researchers are studying how the tumor microenvironment may allow cancer cells to evade immune cells. Immune evasion may result from the abundance of suppressive, regulatory immune cells, excessive inhibitory cytokines, and other features that are not well understood.

Chapter 3

The Respiratory System And How It Works

What Are the Lungs?

Your lungs are organs in your chest that allow your body to take in oxygen from the air. They also help remove carbon dioxide (a waste gas that can be toxic) from your body.

The lungs' intake of oxygen and removal of carbon dioxide is called gas exchange. Gas exchange is part of breathing. Breathing is a vital function of life; it helps your body work properly.

Other organs and tissues also help make breathing possible.

The Respiratory System

The respiratory system is made up of organs and tissues that help you breathe. The main parts of this system are the airways, the lungs and linked blood vessels, and the muscles that enable breathing.

Airways

The airways are pipes that carry oxygen-rich air to your lungs. They also carry carbon dioxide, a waste gas, out of your lungs. The airways include your:

- Nose and linked air passages (called nasal cavities)

- Mouth

About This Chapter: This chapter includes text excerpted from "How The Lungs Work," National Heart, Lung, and Blood Institute (NHLBI), July 17, 2012. Reviewed November 2017.

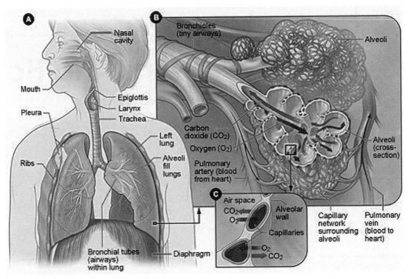

Figure 3.1. The Respiratory System

Figure A shows the location of the respiratory structures in the body. Figure B is an enlarged view of the airways, alveoli (air sacs), and capillaries (tiny blood vessels). Figure C is a closeup view of gas exchange between the capillaries and alveoli. CO2 is carbon dioxide, and O2 is oxygen.

- Larynx, or voice box

- Trachea, or windpipe

- Tubes called bronchial tubes or bronchi, and their branches

Air first enters your body through your nose or mouth, which wets and warms the air. (Cold, dry air can irritate your lungs.) The air then travels through your voice box and down your windpipe. The windpipe splits into two bronchial tubes that enter your lungs.

A thin flap of tissue called the epiglottis covers your windpipe when you swallow. This prevents food and drink from entering the air passages that lead to your lungs.

Except for the mouth and some parts of the nose, all of the airways have special hairs called cilia that are coated with sticky mucus. The cilia trap germs and other foreign particles that enter your airways when you breathe in air.

These fine hairs then sweep the particles up to the nose or mouth. From there, they're swallowed, coughed, or sneezed out of the body. Nose hairs and mouth saliva also trap particles and germs.

Lungs And Blood Vessels

Your lungs and linked blood vessels deliver oxygen to your body and remove carbon dioxide from your body. Your lungs lie on either side of your breastbone and fill the inside of your chest cavity. Your left lung is slightly smaller than your right lung to allow room for your heart.

Within the lungs, your bronchi branch into thousands of smaller, thinner tubes called bronchioles. These tubes end in bunches of tiny round air sacs called alveoli.

Each of these air sacs is covered in a mesh of tiny blood vessels called capillaries. The capillaries connect to a network of arteries and veins that move blood through your body.

The pulmonary artery and its branches deliver blood rich in carbon dioxide (and lacking in oxygen) to the capillaries that surround the air sacs. Inside the air sacs, carbon dioxide moves from the blood into the air. At the same time, oxygen moves from the air into the blood in the capillaries.

The oxygen-rich blood then travels to the heart through the pulmonary vein and its branches. The heart pumps the oxygen-rich blood out to the body.

The lungs are divided into five main sections called lobes. Some people need to have a diseased lung lobe removed. However, they can still breathe well using the rest of their lung lobes.

Muscles Used For Breathing

Muscles near the lungs help expand and contract (tighten) the lungs to allow breathing. These muscles include the:

- Diaphragm
- Intercostal muscles
- Abdominal muscles
- Muscles in the neck and collarbone area

The diaphragm is a dome-shaped muscle located below your lungs. It separates the chest cavity from the abdominal cavity. The diaphragm is the main muscle used for breathing.

The intercostal muscles are located between your ribs. They also play a major role in helping you breathe.

Beneath your diaphragm are abdominal muscles. They help you breathe out when you're breathing fast (for example, during physical activity).

Muscles in your neck and collarbone area help you breathe in when other muscles involved in breathing don't work well, or when lung disease impairs your breathing.

What Happens When You Breathe?

Breathing In (Inhalation)

When you breathe in, or inhale, your diaphragm contracts (tightens) and moves downward. This increases the space in your chest cavity, into which your lungs expand. The intercostal muscles between your ribs also help enlarge the chest cavity. They contract to pull your rib cage both upward and outward when you inhale.

As your lungs expand, air is sucked in through your nose or mouth. The air travels down your windpipe and into your lungs. After passing through your bronchial tubes, the air finally reaches and enters the alveoli (air sacs).

Through the very thin walls of the alveoli, oxygen from the air passes to the surrounding capillaries (blood vessels). A red blood cell protein called hemoglobin helps move oxygen from the air sacs to the blood.

At the same time, carbon dioxide moves from the capillaries into the air sacs. The gas has traveled in the bloodstream from the right side of the heart through the pulmonary artery.

Oxygen-rich blood from the lungs is carried through a network of capillaries to the pulmonary vein. This vein delivers the oxygen-rich blood to the left side of the heart. The left side of the heart pumps the blood to the rest of the body. There, the oxygen in the blood moves from blood vessels into surrounding tissues.

Breathing Out (Exhalation)

When you breathe out, or exhale, your diaphragm relaxes and moves upward into the chest cavity. The intercostal muscles between the ribs also relax to reduce the space in the chest cavity.

As the space in the chest cavity gets smaller, air rich in carbon dioxide is forced out of your lungs and windpipe, and then out of your nose or mouth.

Breathing out requires no effort from your body unless you have a lung disease or are doing physical activity. When you're physically active, your abdominal muscles contract and push your diaphragm against your lungs even more than usual. This rapidly pushes air out of your lungs.

What Controls Your Breathing?

A respiratory control center at the base of your brain controls your breathing. This center sends ongoing signals down your spine and to the muscles involved in breathing.

These signals ensure your breathing muscles contract (tighten) and relax regularly. This allows your breathing to happen automatically, without you being aware of it.

To a limited degree, you can change your breathing rate, such as by breathing faster or holding your breath. Your emotions also can change your breathing. For example, being scared or angry can affect your breathing pattern.

Your breathing will change depending on how active you are and the condition of the air around you. For example, you need to breathe more often when you do physical activity. In contrast, your body needs to restrict how much air you breathe if the air contains irritants or toxins.

To adjust your breathing to changing needs, your body has many sensors in your brain, blood vessels, muscles, and lungs.

Sensors in the brain and in two major blood vessels artery and the aorta) detect carbon dioxide or oxygen levels in your blood and change your breathing rate as needed.

Sensors in the airways detect lung irritants. The sensors can trigger sneezing or coughing. In people who have asthma, the sensors may cause the muscles around the airways in the lungs to contract. This makes the airways smaller.

Sensors in the alveoli (air sacs) can detect fluid buildup in the lung tissues. These sensors are thought to trigger rapid, shallow breathing.

Sensors in your joints and muscles detect movement of your arms or legs. These sensors may play a role in increasing your breathing rate when you're physically active.

Chapter 4

Cold, Flu, Or Allergy?

Know The Difference For Best Treatment

You're feeling pretty lousy. You've got sniffles, sneezing, and a sore throat. Is it a cold, flu, or allergies? It can be hard to tell them apart because they share so many symptoms. But understanding the differences will help you choose the best treatment.

"If you know what you have, you won't take medications that you don't need, that aren't effective, or that might even make your symptoms worse," says National Institutes of Health's (NIH) Dr. Teresa Hauguel, an expert on infectious diseases that affect breathing.

Cold, flu, and allergy all affect your respiratory system, which can make it hard to breathe. Each condition has key symptoms that set them apart.

Colds and flu are caused by different viruses. "As a rule of thumb, the symptoms associated with the flu are more severe," says Hauguel. Both illnesses can lead to a runny, stuffy nose; congestion; cough; and sore throat. But the flu can also cause high fever that lasts for 3—4 days, along with a headache, fatigue, and general aches and pain. These symptoms are less common when you have a cold.

"Allergies are a little different, because they aren't caused by a virus," Hauguel explains. "Instead, it's your body's immune system reacting to a trigger, or allergen, which is something you're allergic to." If you have allergies and breathe in things like pollen or pet dander, the immune cells in your nose and airways may overreact to these harmless substances. Your delicate respiratory tissues may then swell, and your nose may become stuffed up or runny.

About This Chapter: This chapter includes text excerpted from "Cold, Flu, Or Allergy?" *NIH News in Health*, National Institutes of Health (NIH), October 2014. Reviewed November 2017.

"Allergies can also cause itchy, watery eyes, which you don't normally have with a cold or flu," Hauguel adds.

Allergy symptoms usually last as long as you're exposed to the allergen, which may be about 6 weeks during pollen seasons in the spring, summer, or fall. Colds and flu rarely last beyond 2 weeks.

Most people with a cold or flu recover on their own without medical care. But check with a healthcare provider if symptoms last beyond 10 days or if symptoms aren't relieved by over-the-counter medicines.

To treat colds or flu, get plenty of rest and drink lots of fluids. If you have the flu, pain relievers such as aspirin, acetaminophen, or ibuprofen can reduce fever or aches. Allergies can be treated with antihistamines or decongestants.

Be careful to avoid "drug overlap" when taking medicines that list 2 or more active ingredients on the label. For example, if you take 2 different drugs that contain acetaminophen—one for a stuffy nose and the other for headache—you may be getting too much acetaminophen.

Acetaminophen

Acetaminophen is an active ingredient in hundreds of over-the-counter (OTC) and prescription medicines. It relieves pain and fever. And, it is also combined with other active ingredients in medicines that treat allergy, cough, colds, flu, and sleeplessness. In prescription medicines, acetaminophen is found with other active ingredients to treat moderate to severe pain. Acetaminophen can cause serious liver damage if more than directed is used. The U.S. Food and Drug Administration (FDA) has taken action to improve the safety of consumers when using acetaminophen.

(Source: "Acetaminophen Information," U.S. Food and Drug Administration (FDA).)

"Read medicine labels carefully—the warnings, side effects, dosages. If you have questions, talk to your doctor or pharmacist, especially if you have children who are sick," Hauguel says. "You don't want to over medicate, and you don't want to risk taking a medication that may interact with another."

Table 4.1. Allergy And Their Symptoms

Symptoms	Cold	Flu	Airborne Allergy
Fever	Rare	Usual, high (100—102 °F), sometimes higher, especially in young children); lasts 3—4 days	Never
Headache	Uncommon	Common	Uncommon
General Aches, Pains	Slight	Usual; often severe	Never
Fatigue, Weakness	Sometimes	Usual, can last up to 3 weeks	Sometimes
Extreme Exhaustion	Never	Usual, at the beginning of the illness	Never
Stuffy, Runny Nose	Common	Sometimes	Common
Sneezing	Usual	Sometimes	Usual
Sore Throat	Common	Sometimes	Sometimes
Cough	Common	Common, can become severe	Sometimes
Chest Discomfort	Mild to moderate	Common	Rare, except for those with allergic asthma
Treatment	Get plenty of rest. Stay hydrated. (Drink plenty of fluids.) Decongestants. Aspirin (ages 18 and up), acetaminophen, or ibuprofen for aches and pains	Get plenty of rest. Stay hydrated. Aspirin (ages 18 and up), acetaminophen, or ibuprofen for aches, pains, and fever Antiviral medicines (see your doctor)	Avoid allergens (things that you're allergic to) Antihistamines Nasal steroids Decongestants
Prevention	Wash your hands often. Avoid close contact with anyone who has a cold.	Get the flu vaccine each year. Wash your hands often. Avoid close contact with anyone who has the flu.	Avoid allergens, such as pollen, house dust mites, mold, pet dander, cockroaches.
Complications	Sinus infection middle ear infection, asthma	Bronchitis, pneumonia; can be life-threatening	Sinus infection, middle ear infection, asthma

Chapter 5

When You Should See An Allergist

Allergy/immunology is the field of medicine that deals with the human body's immune system. The immune system is a network of cells, tissues, and organs that defends the body against potentially harmful foreign organisms and particles. A physician specializing in this field of medicine is called an allergist/immunologist.

The human body is well equipped to defend itself against disease-causing organisms such as bacteria, viruses, or fungi. It also defends itself from foreign particles such as dust or mold. When the body encounters substances that it recognizes as potentially harmful, the immune system produces antibodies to eliminate them.

Under normal circumstances, this defense mechanism does a good job of protecting the body and keeping it healthy. Sometimes, though, the immune system overreacts to harmless substances—like a certain food or pollen—by releasing chemicals and triggering changes in the body to destroy the invaders. This process is called an allergic reaction. When the reaction is severe enough to require medical care, an allergist/immunologist is usually involved in diagnosing and treating the patient's condition.

Types Of Allergic Reactions

Allergic reactions tend to happen in locations where the immune system has concentrated its defenses to protect against foreign substances entering the body. They frequently affect the skin, the eyes, the respiratory system (nose, sinuses, throat, lungs), and the digestive system (stomach, intestines). Some common types of allergic reactions include contact dermatitis or skin allergies, allergic rhinitis (inflammation of the lining of the nose and sinuses), and asthma.

About This Chapter: "When You Should See An Allergist," © 2015 Omnigraphics. Reviewed November 2017.

Anaphylaxis is a sudden, severe, whole-body allergic reaction that can be life-threatening without immediate medical attention. People can develop allergies to a variety of ordinary substances that they are exposed to daily.

Common types of allergens include: foods such as milk, wheat, nuts, fish, soy, and eggs; airborne particles such as dust, pollen, mold, and pet dander; insect bites and stings; certain chemicals and medications; and substances like latex. Certain plants, like poison ivy, can also trigger severe allergic reactions.

Seeing An Allergist/Immunologist

The symptoms of allergic reactions can range from a mild runny nose or skin rash to diarrhea and vomiting or anaphylaxis. Sometimes the symptoms can be controlled with occasional doses of over-the-counter (OTC) allergy medications, and sometimes they get worse over time and detract from the person's quality of life. Generally speaking, patients should consider seeing an allergist/immunologist under the following circumstances:

- an abnormal reaction to inhaling, ingesting, or coming into contact with something;

- symptoms of asthma such as wheezing, difficulty breathing, or chest pressure;

- more than three infections of the ear, nose, throat, or lungs per year;

- skin conditions like rashes or hives that appear frequently or without a known cause;

- a severe reaction to a bee sting or an insect bite;

- allergic reactions that interfere with performing activities of daily living;

- symptoms that do not improve with the use of over-the-counter medications.

An allergist/immunologist has to undergo a minimum of nine years of medical education and training, including four years of medical school, three years of residency training as an internist or pediatrician, and two years of specialized study in the field of allergy/immunology. The physician then has to pass a certification examination conducted by the American Board of Allergy and Immunology.

An allergist will conduct a medical history and physical examination and perform certain tests to identify the allergen responsible for the patient's reaction. One of the most common tests is the skin-prick test, in which the allergist uses a small needle to prick the patient's skin and insert tiny quantities of allergy-causing substances. If the patient is allergic to a specific substance, they will develop a bump on the skin similar to a mosquito bite. Another test that is often performed by allergists is a challenge test, in which the patient inhales or ingests a very small quantity of allergen under medical supervision to see if they have a reaction. Finally, an allergist may conduct blood tests to check for immunoglobulin E (IgE) antibodies, which are indicators of an allergic reaction.

To prepare for a visit to an allergist, it may be helpful to keep a diary of allergic reactions, recording details about symptoms, exposure to potential allergens, and timing. This information makes it easier for the allergist to diagnose and treat the condition. Prompt diagnosis and identification of allergens will help the patient avoid exposure to these substances or control their reactions if they are exposed to them. Patients with severe allergies may be required to carry emergency medication, like an epinephrine auto-injector or an inhaler, with them at all times.

References

1. "Allergy Testing," American College of Allergy, Asthma, and Immunology, 2015.

2. "When to See an Allergist," American College of Allergy, Asthma, and Immunology, 2014.

Chapter 6

Lung Function Tests For Breathing Problems

Pulmonary function tests, or PFTs, measure how well your lungs work. They include tests that measure lung size and airflow, such as spirometry and lung volume tests. Other tests measure how well gases such as oxygen get in and out of your blood. These tests include pulse oximetry and arterial blood gas tests. Another pulmonary function test, called fractional exhaled nitric oxide (FeNO), measures nitric oxide, which is a marker for inflammation in the lungs. You may have one or more of these tests to diagnose lung and airway diseases, compare your lung function to expected levels of function, monitor if your disease is stable or worsening, and see if your treatment is working.

The purpose, procedure, discomfort, and risks of each test will vary.

- **Spirometry measures the rate of airflow and estimates lung size.** For this test, you will breathe multiple times, with regular and maximal effort, through a tube that is connected to a computer. Some people feel lightheaded or tired from the required breathing effort.

- **Lung volume tests are the most accurate way to measure how much air your lungs can hold.** The procedure is similar to spirometry, except that you will be in a small room with clear walls. Some people feel lightheaded or tired from the required breathing effort.

- **Lung diffusion capacity assesses how well oxygen gets into the blood from the air you breathe.** For this test, you will breathe in and out through a tube for several minutes

---

About This Chapter: Text in this chapter begins with excerpts from "Health Topics—Pulmonary Function Tests," National Heart, Lung, and Blood Institute (NHLBI), December 9, 2016; Text under the heading "Diagnostic Tests And Procedures For Lymphangioleiomyomatosis (LAM)" is excerpted from "LAM—Diagnosis," National Heart, Lung, and Blood Institute (NHLBI), November 15, 2016.

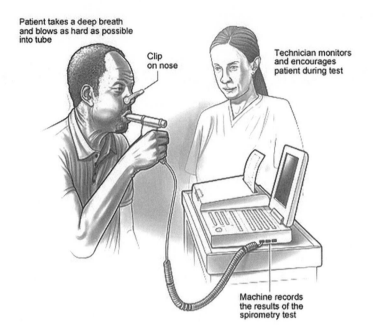

Patient takes a deep breath and blows as hard as possible into tube

Clip on nose

Technician monitors and encourages patient during test

Machine records the results of the spirometry test

Figure 6.1. Spirometry

The image shows how spirometry is done. The patient takes a deep breath and blows as hard as possible into a tube connected to a spirometer. The spirometer measures the amount of air breathed out. It also measures how fast the air was blown out.

(Source: "Explore COPD—Diagnosis," National Heart, Lung, and Blood Institute (NHLBI).)

without having to breathe intensely. You also may need to have blood drawn to measure the level of hemoglobin in your blood.

- **Pulse oximetry estimates oxygen levels in your blood.** For this test, a probe will be placed on your finger or another skin surface such as your ear. It causes no pain and has few or no risks.

- **Arterial blood gas tests directly measure the levels of gases, such as oxygen and carbon dioxide, in your blood.** Arterial blood gas tests are usually performed in a hospital, but may be done in a doctor's office. For this test, blood will be taken from an artery, usually in the wrist where your pulse is measured. You may feel brief pain when the needle is inserted or when a tube attached to the needle fills with blood. It is possible to have bleeding or infection where the needle was inserted.

- **Fractional exhaled nitric oxide tests measure how much nitric oxide is in the air that you exhale.** For this test, you will breathe out into a tube that is connected to the portable device. It requires steady but not intense breathing. It has few or no risks.

Other tests may be needed to assess lung function in infants, children, or patients who are not able to perform spirometry and lung volume tests. Before your tests, you may be asked to not eat some foods or take certain medicines that can affect some pulmonary function test results.

Diagnostic Tests And Procedures For Lymphangioleiomyomatosis (LAM)

Your doctor may recommend tests to show how well your lungs are working and what your lung tissue looks like. These tests can show whether your lungs are delivering enough oxygen to your blood. You also may have tests to check for complications of LAM.

Lung Function Tests

- **Lung function tests.** For lung function tests, you breathe through a mouthpiece into a machine called a spirometer. The spirometer measures the amount of air you breathe in and out. Other lung function tests can show how much air your lungs can hold and how well your lungs deliver oxygen to your blood.

- **Arterial blood gas tests.** Your doctor may take a blood sample from an artery in your wrist to measure your blood oxygen levels and to determine if you need oxygen therapy.

- **Pulse oximetry.** For this test, a small sensor is attached to your finger or ear. The sensor uses light to estimate how much oxygen is in your blood.

- **Six-minute walk test.** This test measures the distance you can walk in six minutes. It can help determine if you need oxygen therapy while exercising.

Imaging Tests

- **Chest X-ray.** A chest X-ray creates a picture of the structures in your chest, such as your heart and lungs. The test can show a collapsed lung or fluid in your chest. In the early stages of LAM, your chest X-rays may look normal. As the disease gets worse, the X-rays may detect cysts in your lungs and assess how cysts change over time.

- **High-resolution CT (HRCT) scan.** The most useful imaging test for diagnosing LAM is a high-resolution CT scan of the chest. This test creates a computer-generated picture of your lungs. The picture shows more detail than the pictures from a chest X-ray. An HRCT scan can show cysts, excess fluid, a collapsed lung, and enlarged lymph nodes. The test also can show how much normal lung tissue has been replaced by the LAM cysts. HRCT scans of your abdomen and pelvis can show whether you have growths in your kidneys, other abdominal organs, or lymph nodes.

Blood Tests For VEGF-D

Your doctor may take a blood sample from a vein in your arm to measure VEGF-D levels. The VEGF-D blood tests test may help confirm the diagnosis of LAM in patients whose HRCT scans show lung cysts that suggest a patient has LAM.

VEGF-D levels of 800 pg/mL (picograms per milliliter) or more can help your doctor confirm that you have LAM. Because you may still have LAM if your levels are less than 800 pg/mL, your doctor may have you undergo other diagnostic procedures that look for LAM cells.

Procedures That Look For LAM Cells

If lung function, imaging, or blood VEGF-D tests cannot diagnose LAM, your doctor may recommend one of the following procedures to collect tissue samples that can be used to detect LAM cells.

- **Video-assisted thoracoscopic surgery (VATS).** In this procedure, your doctor inserts a small, lighted tube into little cuts made in your chest wall. This lets him or her look inside your chest and snip out a few small pieces of lung tissue. VATS is done in a hospital. The procedure isn't major surgery, but it does require general anesthesia to make you sleep during the procedure.

- **Open lung biopsy.** In this procedure, your doctor removes a few small pieces of lung tissue through a cut made in your chest wall between your ribs. An open lung biopsy is done in a hospital. You'll be given medicine to make you sleep during the procedure. Open lung biopsies are rarely done anymore because the recovery time is much longer than the recovery time from VATS.

- **Transbronchial biopsy.** In this procedure, your doctor inserts a long, narrow, flexible, lighted tube down your windpipe and into your lungs. He or she then snips out bits of lung tissue using a tiny device. This procedure usually is done in a hospital. Your mouth and throat are numbed to prevent pain. Because only a small amount of tissue is collected, it is possible that this test will not provide enough information.

- **Other biopsies.** Your doctor also can diagnose LAM using the results from other tissue biopsies, such as biopsies of lymph nodes or abdominal or pelvic lesions.

Other Tests

If your chest imaging tests show that you have pleural effusions, your doctor may order a pleural fluid analysis. For this test, a fluid sample is taken from the pleural space, which is a thin space between two layers of tissue that line the lungs and chest cavity. Doctors use a procedure called thoracentesis to collect the fluid sample. The fluid is studied for the milky substance called chylothorax.

If you're diagnosed with sporadic LAM, your doctor may advise you to have a computed tomography (CT) scan or magnetic resonance imaging (MRI) scan of your head. These tests can help screen for underlying tuberous sclerosis complex (TSC), a condition that can also cause kidney growths and lung cysts. If a woman who has cysts in her lungs is found to have TSC, the doctor will diagnose TSC-associated LAM or TSC–LAM.

Chapter 7

Patch Tests For Allergies

What Is Allergen Patch Tests?

Allergen patch tests are diagnostic tests applied to the surface of the skin. Patch tests are used by healthcare providers to determine the specific cause of contact dermatitis, and are manufactured from natural substances or chemicals (such as nickel, rubber, and fragrance mixes) that are known to cause contact dermatitis.

Indications And Usage

T.R.U.E. TEST® is an epicutaneous patch test indicated for use as an aid in the diagnosis of allergic contact dermatitis (ACD) in persons 6 years of age and older whose history suggests sensitivity to one or more of the 35 allergens and allergen mixes included on the T.R.U.E. TEST panels.

Dosage And Administration

Dose

T.R.U.E. TEST contains three adhesive panels consisting of 35 allergen and allergen mix patches and a 15 negative control.

About This Chapter: This chapter includes text excerpted from "Allergenics—Allergen Patch Tests," Child Welfare Information Gateway, U.S. Food and Drug Administration (FDA), March 7, 2017.

Administration

Application Instructions

T.R.U.E. TEST should only be applied to healthy skin. Test sites should be free of scars, acne, dermatitis, or other conditions that may interfere with test result interpretation. Avoid application of T.R.U.E. TEST panels to tanned or sun exposed skin because this may increase the risk of false negatives. Avoid patch testing for three (3) weeks after ultraviolet (UV) treatments, heavy sun, or tanning bed exposure. Avoid using alcohol or other irritating substances on the skin prior to testing. Avoid excessive sweating during the testing period to maintain sufficient adhesion to the skin. Avoid excessive physical activity to maintain sufficient adhesion and to prevent actual loss of patch test material. Avoid getting the panels and surrounding area wet. If excessive body hair exists at the test site, remove with an electric shaver (do not use razors). Very oily skin may be cleaned with mild soap and water prior to testing.

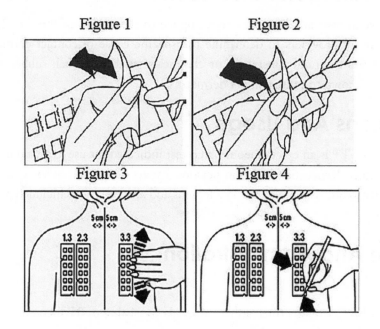

Figure 7.1. T.R.U.E. Test Procedure

Test panels should be applied as follows:

1. Peel open the package and remove the test panel (Figure 1).

2. Remove the protective plastic covering from the test surface of the panel (Figure 2). Be careful not to touch the test allergens or allergen mixes.

3. Position test Panel 1.3 on the patient's back as shown in Figure 3. Allergen number 1 should be in the upper left corner. Avoid applying the panel on the margin of the scapula or directly over the midline of the spine. Ensure that each patch of the allergen panel is in contact with the skin by smoothing the panel outward from the center to the edge (as illustrated for Panel 3.3 in Figure 3).

4. With a medical marking pen, indicate on the skin the location of the two notches on the panel (as illustrated for Panel 3.3 in Figure 4).

5. Repeat the process with test Panel 2.3. Position the test Panel 2.3 beside Panel 1.3, on the left side of the patient's back so that the number 13 allergen is in the upper left corner. Apply test Panel 2.3 five (5) cm from the midline of the spine (Figure 3).

6. Repeat the process with Panel 3.3 positioning the panel on the right side of the patient's back so that the number 25 allergen is in the upper left corner. Apply test Panel 3.3 five (5) cm from the midline of 54 the spine. (Figure 3)

7. If needed, hypoallergenic surgical tape, appropriate for patch testing, may be used for increased adhesion around the outside edges of the panels.

Timing Of Test Readings

Patients are scheduled to return approximately 48 hours after patch test application to have the panels removed. Prior to removal of the panels, use a medical marking pen to remark the notches found on the panels. The patch test reaction on the patient's skin may be evaluated at 48 hours, but an additional reading(s) at 72 and/or 96 hours is necessary. Late positive reactions may occur 7 to 21 days after application of the panels.

Interpretation Instructions

An identification template is provided for each of the three (3) panels for quick identification of any allergen that causes a reaction. To assure correct positioning, marks on the skin made with the medical marking pen should correlate with the notches on the template. The interpretation method, similar to the one recommended by the International Contact Dermatitis Research Group, is as follows:

- ? Doubtful reaction: faint macular erythema only

- + Weak positive reaction: nonvesicular with erythema, infiltration, possibly papules

- ++ Strong positive reaction: vesicular, erythema, infiltration, papules

- +++ Extreme positive reaction: bullous or ulcerative reaction

- – Negative reaction

- IR Irritant reaction: Pustules as well as patchy follicular or homogeneous erythema without infiltrations are usually signs of irritation and do not indicate allergy.

Itching is a subjective symptom that is expected to accompany a positive reaction.

False Negatives

False negative results may be due to insufficient patch contact with the skin and/or premature evaluation of the test. Repeat testing may be indicated. The effect of repetitive testing with T.R.U.E. TEST is unknown.

False Positives

A false positive result may occur when an irritant reaction cannot be differentiated from an allergic reaction. A positive test reaction should meet the criteria for an allergic reaction. If an irritant reaction cannot be distinguished from a true positive reaction or if a doubtful reaction is present, a retest may be considered. The effect of repetitive testing with T.R.U.E. TEST is unknown.

Chapter 8

Allergy Blood Test

What Is An Allergy Blood Test?

Allergies are a common and chronic condition that involves the body's immune system. Normally, your immune system works to fight off viruses, bacteria, and other infectious agents. When you have an allergy, your immune system treats a harmless substance, like dust or pollen, as a threat. To fight this perceived threat, your immune system makes antibodies called immunoglobulin E (IgE).

Substances that cause an allergic reaction are called allergens. Besides dust and pollen, other common allergens include animal dander, foods, including nuts and shellfish, and certain medicines, such as penicillin. Allergy symptoms can range from sneezing and a stuffy nose to a life-threatening complication called anaphylactic shock. Allergy blood tests measure the amount of IgE antibodies in the blood. A small amount of IgE antibodies is normal. A larger amount of IgE may mean you have an allergy.

Other Names
IgE allergy test, Quantitative IgE, Immunoglobulin E, Total IgE, Specific IgE

What Is It Used For?

Allergy blood tests are used to find out if you have an allergy. One type of test called a total IgE test measures the overall number of IgE antibodies in your blood. Another type of

About This Chapter: This chapter includes text excerpted from "Allergy Blood Test," MedlinePlus, National Institutes of Health (NIH), September 6, 2017.

allergy blood test called a specific IgE test measures the level of IgE antibodies in response to individual allergens.

Why Do I Need An Allergy Blood Test?

Your healthcare provider may order allergy testing if you have symptoms of an allergy. These include:

- Stuffy or runny nose
- Sneezing
- Itchy, watery eyes
- Hives (a rash with raised red patches)
- Diarrhea
- Vomiting
- Shortness of breath
- Coughing
- Wheezing

What Happens During An Allergy Blood Test?

A healthcare professional will take a blood sample from a vein in your arm, using a small needle. After the needle is inserted, a small amount of blood will be collected into a test tube or vial. You may feel a little sting when the needle goes in or out. This usually takes less than five minutes.

Will I Need To Do Anything To Prepare For The Test?

You don't need any special preparations for an allergy blood test.

Are There Any Risks To The Test?

There is very little risk to having an allergy blood test. You may have slight pain or bruising at the spot where the needle was put in, but most symptoms go away quickly.

What Do The Results Mean?

If your total IgE levels are higher than normal, it likely means you have some kind of allergy. But it does not reveal what you are allergic to. A specific IgE test will help identify your particular allergy. If your results indicate an allergy, your healthcare provider may refer you to an allergy specialist or recommend a treatment plan.

Your treatment plan will depend on the type and severity of your allergy. People at risk for anaphylactic shock, a severe allergic reaction that can cause death, need to take extra care to avoid the allergy causing substance. They may need to carry an emergency epinephrine treatment with them at all times.

Be sure to talk to your healthcare provider if you have questions about your test results and/ or your allergy treatment plan.

Is There Anything Else I Need To Know About An Allergy Blood Test?

An IgE skin test is another way to detect allergies, by measuring IgE levels and looking for a reaction directly on the skin. Your healthcare provider may order an IgE skin test instead of, or in addition to, an IgE allergy blood test.

Chapter 9

Allergy Shots (Immunotherapy)

Children are magnets for colds. But when the sniffles and sneezing won't go away for weeks, the culprit may be allergies.

Long-lasting sneezing, with a stuffy or runny nose, may signal the presence of allergic rhinitis—the collection of symptoms that affect the nose when you have an allergic reaction to something you breathe in and that lands on the lining inside the nose.

Allergies may be seasonal or can strike year round (perennial). In most parts of the United States, plant pollens are often the cause of seasonal allergic rhinitis—more commonly called hay fever. Indoor substances, such as mold, dust mites, and pet dander, may cause the perennial kind.

Up to 40 percent of children suffer from allergic rhinitis. And children are more likely to develop allergies if one or both parents have allergies.

The U.S. Food and Drug Administration (FDA) regulates over-the-counter (OTC) and prescription medicines that offer allergy relief as well as allergen extracts used to diagnose and treat allergies. Take care to read and follow the directions provided when giving any medicine to children, including these products.

About This Chapter: Text in this chapter begins with excerpts from "For Consumers—Allergy Relief For Your Child," U.S. Food and Drug Administration (FDA), June 1, 2017; Text beginning with the heading "What Are Allergy Shots And Allergy Drops?" is excerpted from "Allergy Shots And Allergy Drops For Adults And Children," Agency for Healthcare Research and Quality (AHRQ), U.S. Department of Health and Human Services (HHS), August 2013. Reviewed November 2017.

Immune System Reaction

An allergy is the body's reaction to a specific substance, or allergen. Our immune system responds to the invading allergen by releasing histamine and other chemicals that typically trigger symptoms in the nose, lungs, throat, sinuses, ears, eyes, skin, or stomach lining.

In some children, allergies can also trigger symptoms of asthma—a disease that causes wheezing or difficulty breathing. If a child has allergies and asthma, "not controlling the allergies can make asthma worse," says Anthony Durmowicz, M.D., a pediatric pulmonary doctor at the FDA.

Avoid Pollen, Mold, And Other Allergy Triggers

If the child has seasonal allergies, pay attention to pollen counts and try to keep the child inside when the levels are high.

- In the late summer and early fall, during ragweed pollen season, pollen levels are highest in the morning.

- In the spring and summer, during the grass pollen season, pollen levels are highest in the evening.

- Some molds, another allergy trigger, may also be seasonal. For example, leaf mold is more common in the fall.

- Sunny, windy days can be especially troublesome for pollen allergy sufferers.

It may also help to keep windows closed in your house and car and run the air conditioner.

Allergy Medicines For Children

For most children, symptoms may be controlled by avoiding the allergen, if known, and using OTC medicines. But if a child's symptoms are persistent and not relieved by OTC medicines, see a healthcare professional.

Although some allergy medicines are approved for use in children as young as 6 months, the FDA cautions that simply because a product's box says that it is intended for children does not mean it is intended for children of all ages. Always read the label to make sure the product is right for the child's age.

When the child is taking more than one medication, read the label to be sure that the active ingredients aren't the same. Although the big print may say the product is to treat a certain symptom, different products may have the same medicine (active ingredient). It might seem that you are buying different products to treat different symptoms, but in fact the same medicine could be in all the products. The result: You might accidentally be giving too much of one type of medicine to the child.

Children are more sensitive than adults to many drugs. For example, some antihistamines can have adverse effects at lower doses on young patients, causing excitability or excessive drowsiness.

Allergy Shots And Children

Jay E. Slater, M.D., a pediatric allergist at the FDA, says that children who don't respond to either OTC or prescription medications, or who suffer from frequent complications of allergic rhinitis, may be candidates for allergen immunotherapy—commonly known as allergy shots.

Immunotherapy (SCIT), as a treatment for allergic diseases, was first introduced by Noon and Freeman in 1911 as a means of treating grass-induced allergic symptomatology "hay fever" (i.e., rhinoconjunctivitis).

(Source: "Allergen-Specific Immunotherapy For The Treatment Of Allergic Rhinoconjunctivitis And/ Or Asthma," Agency for Healthcare Research and Quality (AHRQ), U.S. Department of Health and Human Services (HHS).)

After allergy testing, typically by skin testing to detect what allergens the child may react to, a healthcare professional injects the child with "extracts"—small amounts of the allergens that trigger a reaction. The doses are gradually increased so that the body builds up immunity to these allergens. Allergen extracts are manufactured from natural substances, such as pollens, insect venoms, animal hair, and foods. More than 1,200 extracts are licensed by the FDA.

In 2014, the FDA approved three new immunotherapy products that are taken under the tongue for treatment of hay fever caused by certain pollens, two of them for use in children. All of them are intended for daily use, before and during the pollen season. They are not meant for immediate symptom relief. Although they are intended for at home use, these are prescription medications, and first doses are taken in the presence of a healthcare provider.

In 2017, the FDA approved Odactra, the first immunotherapy product administered under the tongue for treatment of house dust mite induced allergic rhinitis (nasal inflammation) with or without conjunctivitis (eye inflammation). Odactra is approved for use only in adults.

"Allergy shots are never appropriate for food allergies," adds Slater, "but it's common to use extracts to test for food allergies so the child can avoid those foods."

"In the last 20 years, there has been a remarkable transformation in allergy treatments," says Slater. "Kids used to be miserable for months out of the year, and drugs made them incredibly sleepy. But today's products offer proven approaches for relief of seasonal allergy symptoms."

What Are Allergy Shots And Allergy Drops?

Allergy shots and allergy drops help your immune system become less sensitive to allergens. The shots and drops contain a tiny amount of the allergens that cause your allergies. For example, if you are allergic to oak tree pollen, your shots or drops will have a tiny amount of oak tree pollen in them. Allergy shots and drops both contain the allergens that cause your allergies. The difference between them is simply in how they are given. The amount of the allergen in allergy shots or drops is so small that your immune system likely will not react strongly to it. Your doctor will talk with you about what to do if you have a strong reaction. Your doctor will slowly put more of the allergen into your shots or drops until your immune system becomes less sensitive to the allergen. This means your immune system will not react strongly when you breathe in the allergen. Over time, your immune system will start to tolerate the allergen, and your allergy symptoms will get better.

Some people may not be able to take allergy shots or drops. You should talk with your doctor if:

- You (or your child) have severe asthma
- You (or your child) take a type of medicine called a "beta blocker," used to treat high blood pressure
- You (or your child) have heart problems
- You are pregnant or are thinking of becoming pregnant
- You are considering allergy shots or allergy drops for a child under 5 years of age.

Table 9.1. Comparing Allergy Shots And Allergy Drops

	Allergy Shots	**Allergy Drops**
How are they taken?	The shots are given under the skin (often in the upper arm) usually at the doctor's office.	The liquid drops are placed under the tongue and are usually taken at home

Table 9.1. Continued

	Allergy Shots	Allergy Drops
How often do you take them?	One or more shots each time you go to the doctor's office: • Once or twice a week for the first few months • Once or twice a month after that	A few times a week or every day
How long do you take them?	3 to 5 years (or sometimes longer)	3 to 5 years (or sometimes longer) Typically 3 to 5 years (or sometimes longer)
Are they approved by the U.S. Food and Drug Administration (FDA) to treat allergies and asthma caused by allergies?	Yes	No, allergy drops are not yet approved by the FDA.* But they are approved and commonly used in Europe and other parts of the world. Allergy drops are available in the United States, and doctors are starting to prescribe them

Because allergy drops are not yet approved by the FDA, they may not be covered by your health insurance.

What Have Researchers Found About How Well Allergy Shots And Allergy Drops Work?

In adults:

• Both allergy shots and allergy drops improve allergy and mild asthma symptoms.

• Both allergy shots and allergy drops lessen the need to take allergy and asthma medicines.

• Both allergy shots and allergy drops improve quality of life.

In children:

• Both allergy shots and allergy drops improve allergy and mild asthma symptoms.

• Allergy drops lessen the need to take allergy and asthma medicines.

• Allergy shots also appear to lessen the need to take allergy and asthma medicines, but more research is needed to know this for sure.

Researchers also found:

- There is not enough research to know if allergy shots or allergy drops work better.

Nearly 80 percent of peanut-allergic preschool children successfully incorporated peanut-containing foods into their diets after receiving peanut oral immunotherapy (OIT), a clinical trial has found. Peanut OIT involves eating small, gradually increasing amounts of peanut protein daily. Low-dose and high-dose OIT were safe and equally effective at suppressing allergic immune responses to peanut, investigators found. The work was partly supported by the National Institute of Allergy and Infectious Diseases (NIAID) and the National Center for Advancing Translational Sciences, both part of the National Institutes of Health (NIH).

(Source: "Oral Immunotherapy Is Safe, Effective Treatment For Peanut-Allergic Preschoolers, Study Suggests," National Institute of Allergy and Infectious Diseases (NIAID).)

What Are The Possible Side Effects Of Allergy Shots And Allergy Drops?

Allergy shots and allergy drops are safe, and side effects are usually mild.

Common side effects of allergy shots include:

- Itching, swelling, and redness at the place where the shot was given
- Headache
- Coughing
- Tiredness
- Mucus dripping down your throat
- Sneezing

Common side effects of allergy drops include:

- Throat irritation
- Itching or mild swelling in the mouth

Although it is rare, allergy shots and allergy drops could cause a life-threatening allergic reaction called "anaphylaxis." Symptoms of anaphylaxis can include severe swelling of the face, throat, or tongue; itching; a skin rash; trouble breathing; tightness in the chest; wheezing; dizziness; nausea; diarrhea; or loss of consciousness. If you or your child has any of these symptoms after getting an allergy shot or taking allergy drops, call the doctor right away. Anaphylaxis must be treated immediately with a shot of epinephrine, a type of hormone that regulates your heart rate and breathing passages.

What Are The Costs Of Allergy Shots And Allergy Drops?

The costs to you for allergy shots and allergy drops depend on your health insurance. Because allergy drops are not yet approved by the U.S. Food and Drug Administration (FDA), they may not be covered by your health insurance. The costs also depend on how many allergens are in your allergy shots or allergy drops. Because allergy shots are usually given at the doctor's office, you may have to pay for an office visit each time you go for a shot.

What Should I Think About When Deciding?

There are many things to think about when deciding if allergy shots or allergy drops are right for you or your child. You may want to talk with your doctor about:

- How severe your (or your child's) allergy or asthma symptoms are

- How well you are able to avoid or reduce allergens in your environment (for example, cleaning carpets and drapes or using an air filter, mattress cover, or special pillow case)

- How well allergy medicines (antihistamines or steroid nasal spray) work to improve your (or your child's) symptoms

- Possible benefits and side effects of allergy shots or allergy drops

- Which might work better to improve your (or your child's) allergy or asthma symptoms—allergy shots or allergy drops

- Which better fits your preferences and lifestyle—allergy shots or allergy drops For example, would it be easier to take allergy drops every day or go to the doctor's office every few days for a shot?

- The costs of allergy shots or allergy drops

Ask Your Doctor

- What are the best ways for me to avoid or reduce allergens in my environment?

- Could allergy shots or drops help me (or my child)?

- Do any of my (or my child's) medical conditions affect my (or my child's) ability to take allergy shots or allergy drops?

- Which do you think would be better—allergy shots or allergy drops?

- How long will it take for the allergy shots or allergy drops to start helping?

- How long will I (or my child) need to take the allergy shots or allergy drops?

- How long will allergy shots or allergy drops improve my (or my child's) allergy or asthma symptoms?

- How much would allergy shots cost? How much would allergy drops cost?

- Are there side effects that I need to call you about right away or that would require me to go to an emergency room? If so, what are they? What should I do? When are they likely to happen?

Chapter 10

Medications Used To Treat Allergic Symptoms

The pollen count is sky high. You're sneezing, your eyes are itching, and you feel miserable. Seasonal allergies are real diseases that can interfere with work, school or recreation. Allergies can also trigger or worsen asthma and lead to other health problems such as sinus infection (sinusitis) and ear infections in children.

An allergy is your body's reaction to a substance that it has identified as an invader. If you have allergies and encounter a trigger—called an "allergen"—your immune system fights it by releasing chemicals called histamines (hence the term "antihistamines"). Histamines cause symptoms such as repetitive sneezing and itchy, watery eyes.

Allergy Medicines: Antihistamines And More

Seasonal allergies are usually caused by plant pollen, which can come from trees, weeds and grasses in the spring, and by ragweed and other weeds in late summer and early fall.

Since you can't always stay indoors when pollen counts are high, your healthcare provider may recommend prescription or over-the-counter (OTC) medications to relieve symptoms. The U.S. Food and Drug Administration (FDA) regulates a number of medications that offer allergy relief.

Antihistamines reduce or block symptom causing histamines and are available in many forms, including tablets and liquids. Many oral antihistamines are available OTC and in generic form.

About This Chapter: Text in this chapter begins with excerpts from "For Consumers—Seasonal Allergies: Which Medication Is Right For You?" U.S. Food and Drug Administration (FDA), June 1, 2017; Text under the heading "Leukotriene Receptor Antagonists" is excerpted from "Drug Record—Leukotriene Receptor Antagonists," LiverTox®, National Institutes of Health (NIH), October 16, 2017.

When choosing an OTC antihistamine, patients should read the Drug Facts label closely and follow dosing instructions, says Jenny Kelty, M.D., a pediatric pulmonologist at the FDA. Some antihistamines can cause drowsiness and interfere with the ability to drive or operate heavy machinery, like a car. There are other antihistamines that do not have this side effect; they are nonsedating. Some nonsedating antihistamines are available by prescription.

Nasal corticosteroids are typically sprayed into the nose once or twice a day to treat inflammation. Side effects may include stinging in the nose.

Decongestants are drugs available both by prescription and OTC and come in oral and nasal spray forms. They are sometimes recommended in combination with antihistamines, which used alone do not have an effect on nasal congestion.

Drugs that contain pseudoephedrine are available without a prescription but are kept behind the pharmacy counter to prevent their use in making methamphetamine—a powerful, highly addictive stimulant often produced illegally in home laboratories. You will need to ask your pharmacist and show identification to purchase drugs that contain pseudoephedrine.

Using decongestant nose sprays and drops more than a few days may give you a "rebound" effect—your nasal congestion could get worse. These drugs are more useful for short-term use to relieve nasal congestion.

Immunotherapy may help if other medications don't relieve your symptoms. One form of allergen immunotherapy is allergy shots in which your body responds to injected amounts of a particular allergen, given in gradually increasing doses, by developing immunity or tolerance to that allergen.

Multiple allergen immunotherapies can be defined as the use of extracts containing more than one allergen class, whereas single allergen immunotherapy can refer to the use of closely related allergens within the same class. For example, a study using a grass mix allergen (or tree mix, or 2 dust mite species) could be considered a single allergen study, whereas a multiple allergen study could use different classes of allergens, such as tree and grass.

(Source: "Allergen-Specific Immunotherapy For The Treatment Of Allergic Rhinoconjunctivitis And/ Or Asthma," Agency for Healthcare Research and Quality (AHRQ), U.S. Department of Health and Human Services (HHS).)

Patients can receive injections from a healthcare provider; a common course of treatment would begin with weekly injections for two to three months until the maximum dose is reached. After that, treatment could continue monthly for three to five years.

Another form of allergen immunotherapy therapy involves administering the allergens in a tablet form under the tongue (sublingual) and are intended for daily use, before and during the pollen season. These medications have the potential for dialing down the immune response to allergens and are not meant for immediate symptom relief, says Kelty. Sublingual therapy should start three to four months before allergy season. Although they are intended for at home use, these are prescription medications, and the first doses are to be taken in the presence of a healthcare provider.

Leukotriene Receptor Antagonists

The leukotriene receptor antagonists (LTRAs) are among the most prescribed drugs for the management of asthma, used both for treatment and prevention of acute asthmatic attacks. This class of drugs acts by binding to cysteinyl leukotriene (CysLT) receptors and blocking their activation and the subsequent inflammatory cascade which cause the symptoms commonly associated with asthma and allergic rhinitis.

The cysteinyl leukotrienes (C4, D4 and E4) are products of arachidonic acid metabolism and are released from various cells, including mast cells and eosinophils. These eicosanoids bind to CysLT receptors. The CysLT type-1 receptor is found in the human airway smooth muscle cells and airway macrophages and on other proinflammatory cells. In asthmatic patients, leukotriene mediated effects include airway edema, smooth muscle contraction, and altered cellular activity associated with the inflammatory process. In allergic rhinitis, CysLTs are released from the nasal mucosa after allergen exposure and precipitate the symptoms of allergic rhinitis.

Two leukotriene receptor antagonists are available in the United States, zafirlukast (1996) and montelukast (1998). Both are oral agents used in management of asthma and allergic rhinitis. Both have been associated with rare cases of acute liver injury. While they have similar mechanisms of action, these two agents are structurally distinct, and the liver injury they cause does not appear to be similar in pattern of presentation or outcome.

A Word About OTC Products And Kids

Always read the label before buying an OTC product for you or your children, says Kelty. "Some products can be used in children as young as 2 years, but others are not appropriate for children of any age." Talk to your healthcare professional if your child needs to use nasal steroid spray for more than two months a year.

Chapter 11

Epinephrine Injections For Life-Threatening Allergic Reactions

What Are Epinephrine Injections?

Epinephrine injections are used to treat severe allergic reactions or anaphylaxis. Insect bites or stings, food, latex, medicines, or other allergens can cause life-threatening allergic reactions that require immediate medical treatment. The chemical epinephrine helps relax airways and narrows blood vessels to reverse wheezing, hives, skin itching, severe low blood pressure, and other serious allergic reactions. The medication is only available with a doctor's prescription and can be ordered in injectable or solution form. For individuals with a history of allergic attacks, epinephrine is most conveniently available in an auto-injector.

How Should Epinephrine Injections Be Used?

Epinephrine injections should always be used under the direction of a qualified healthcare provider. The needle or prefilled automatic injection device can be inserted under the skin or into the muscle, most often into the thigh. Injecting into the hands or feet is not recommended, since this can cause side effects resulting in reduced blood flow to those regions. Young children may squirm or flinch when being given an injection, so it's important to hold their legs firmly in position before and after the shot. After use, some residue may remain in the injector, which is normal, but this liquid should not be reused.

About This Chapter: "Epinephrine Injections For Life-Threatening Allergic Reactions," © 2017 Omnigraphics. Reviewed November 2017.

Using An Epinephrine Auto-Injector

An epinephrine auto-injector contains a needle kit and the exact dosage of medicine prescribed by a doctor. The device can be used only once and needs to be discarded properly after use. Here are the steps for using an epinephrine auto-injector:

- The auto-injector comes with a safety cap that should not be removed until the patient is ready to use it. To remove the safety cap, grasp the injector with its tip pointing down and pull off the cap.

- To avoid accidental injection, keep fingers away from the tip while removing the cap.

- After removal of the safety cap, place the auto-injector tip on the thigh.

- Inject the dose into the thigh muscle by pushing on the auto-injector, which will release the needle and deliver the medication. Hold the auto-injector in place for about 10 seconds.

- After the injection, remove the auto-injector, and gently massage the area.

- Re-cap the device and place it into its carrying tube. Then take it to the healthcare provider, who will record how much epinephrine has been used and dispose of the injector properly.

Precautions About The Use Of Epinephrine Injections

A number of precautions must be taken while using epinephrine injections, especially if the patient needs to use the medication frequently:

- Be sure to inject doses at regular time intervals as prescribed by a healthcare provider.

- The medication should never be injected into the buttocks muscle or into a vein.

- If a family member is helping the patient with epinephrine injections, that individual needs to understand how to administrate the drug properly.

- To avoid accidental injection, the safety release or end caps should not be removed prior to use.

- Epinephrine auto-injectors come with a "trainer pen," which contains no medicine or needle. The trainer pen is used for practice so that the patient or caregiver can be prepared before an emergency.

- The effects of the medication generally last from 10 to 20 minutes, and since epinephrine is only a first line of treatment, further observation and consultation with a medical professional is required.

- If the patient does not respond to the first shot of epinephrine, then a second dose could be administered, but only under medical supervision.

- Patients who are prone to allergic reactions should always carry an epinephrine injector with them.

- If the liquid changes color, or if there are solids present in it, the medication should be discarded. Regularly checking the liquid for discoloration or other signs of deterioration is essential.

- The medicine needs to be kept at normal temperature; it should not be refrigerated or allowed to be in direct sunlight or heat.

- The expired medicine should be discarded properly.

- The injection should be kept out of children's reach. They should never be allowed to use it on their own.

- Dosages differ from person to person. The dosage should not be changed by the patient unless advised by a healthcare provider.

Discussion With A Healthcare Provider Before Using Epinephrine Injections

A healthcare provider needs to know the detailed health condition of a patient before prescribing epinephrine injections. The following are some of the topics that will be covered:

- If the patient is allergic to sulfites or to any medications.

- All the prescribed and over-the-counter (OTC) medicines the patient is currently taking.

- Whether the patient has associated illnesses, such as Parkinson disease, asthma, diabetes, heart disease, high blood pressure, hyperthyroidism, depression, or irregular heartbeat.

- If the patient is pregnant or breastfeeding.

Side Effects Of Epinephrine Injection

Some common side effects include pounding heartbeats, dizziness, feeling weak or tired, pale skin, shivering, headache, or vomiting. If the patient experiences certain side effects like redness of the skin, infection around the injection site, swelling, pain, or warmth, a healthcare provider should be contacted immediately.

Symptoms Of Epinephrine Injection Overdose

An overdose can cause symptoms such as shortness of breath, sudden numbness or paralysis on one side of the body, cold or pale skin, decreased urination, fast breathing, unusually slow or fast heart rate, difficulty with speech, and confusion. Immediate medical attention is required if these symptoms are present.

References

1. "Epinephrine Injection," U.S. National Library of Medicine, September 21, 2017.

2. "Epinephrine (Injection Route)," Mayo Clinic, March 1, 2017.

3. "Epinephrine Injection," Drugs.com, September 1, 2017.

4. Wood, Joseph P., MD, Stephen J. Traub, MD, and Christopher Lipinski, MD. "Safety of Epinephrine for Anaphylaxis in the Emergency Setting," National Library of Medicine (NLM), 2013.

Part Two
Allergy Symptoms And Complications

Chapter 12

Coughing And Sneezing

What Is Cough?

A cough is a natural reflex that protects your lungs. Coughing helps clear your airways of lung irritants, such as smoke and mucus (a slimy substance). This helps prevent infections. A cough also can be a symptom of a medical problem. Prolonged coughing can cause unpleasant side effects, such as chest pain, exhaustion, light-headedness, and loss of bladder control. Coughing also can interfere with sleep, socializing, and work.

What Causes Cough?

Coughing occurs when the nerve endings in your airways become irritated. Certain irritants and allergens, medical conditions, and medicines can irritate these nerve endings.

Irritants And Allergens

An irritant is something you're sensitive to. For example, smoking or inhaling secondhand smoke can irritate your lungs. Smoking also can lead to medical conditions that can cause a cough. Other irritants include air pollution, paint fumes, or scented products like perfumes or air fresheners.

An allergen is something you're allergic to, such as dust, animal dander, mold, or pollens from trees, grasses, and flowers.

Coughing helps clear your airways of irritants and allergens. This helps prevent infections.

About This Chapter: This chapter includes text excerpted from "Cough," National Heart, Lung, and Blood Institute (NHLBI), June 11, 2014. Reviewed November 2017.

Medical Conditions

Many medical conditions can cause acute, subacute, or chronic cough. Common causes of an acute cough are a common cold, or other upper respiratory infections. Examples of other upper respiratory infections include the flu, pneumonia, and whooping cough. An acute cough lasts less than 3 weeks.

A lingering cough that remains after a cold or other respiratory infection is gone often is called a subacute cough. A subacute cough lasts 3 to 8 weeks.

Common causes of a chronic cough are upper airway cough syndrome (UACS), asthma, and gastroesophageal reflux disease (GERD). A chronic cough lasts more than 8 weeks.

"UACS" is a term used to describe conditions that inflame the upper airways and cause a cough. Examples include sinus infections and allergies. These conditions can cause mucus (a slimy substance) to run down your throat from the back of your nose. This is called postnasal drip.

Asthma is a long-term lung disease that inflames and narrows the airways. GERD is a condition in which acid from your stomach backs up into your throat.

Other conditions that can cause a chronic cough include:

- **Respiratory infections.** A cough from an upper respiratory infection can develop into a chronic cough.
- **Chronic bronchitis.** This condition occurs if the lining of the airways is constantly irritated and inflamed. Smoking is the main cause of chronic bronchitis.
- **Bronchiectasis.** This is a condition in which damage to the airways causes them to widen and become flabby and scarred. This prevents the airways from properly moving mucus out of your lungs. An infection or other condition that injures the walls of the airways usually causes bronchiectasis.
- **COPD (chronic obstructive pulmonary disease).** COPD is a disease that prevents enough air from flowing in and out of the airways.
- **Lung cancer.** In rare cases, a chronic cough is due to lung cancer. Most people who develop lung cancer smoke or used to smoke.
- **Heart failure.** Heart failure is a condition in which the heart can't pump enough blood to meet the body's needs. Fluid can buildup in the body and lead to many symptoms. If fluid builds up in the lungs, it can cause a chronic cough.

Medicines

Certain medicines can cause a chronic cough. Examples of these medicines are angiotensin-converting-enzyme (ACE) inhibitors and beta blockers. ACE inhibitors are used to treat high blood pressure (HBP). Beta blockers are used to treat HBP, migraine headaches, and glaucoma.

Who Is At Risk For Cough?

People at risk for cough include those who:

- Are exposed to things that irritate their airways (called irritants) or things that they're allergic to (called allergens). Examples of irritants are cigarette smoke, air pollution, paint fumes, and scented products. Examples of allergens are dust, animal dander, mold, and pollens from trees, grasses, and flowers.

- Have certain conditions that irritate the lungs, such as asthma, sinus infections, colds, or gastroesophageal reflux disease.

- Smoke. Smoking can irritate your lungs and cause coughing. Smoking and/or exposure to secondhand smoke also can lead to medical conditions that can cause a cough.

- Take certain medicines, such as ACE inhibitors and beta blockers. ACE inhibitors are used to treat high blood pressure (HBP). Beta blockers are used to treat HBP, migraine headaches, and glaucoma.

What Are The Signs And Symptoms Of Cough?

When you cough, mucus (a slimy substance) may come up. Coughing helps clear the mucus in your airways from a cold, bronchitis, or other condition. Rarely, people cough up blood. If this happens, you should call your doctor right away.

A cough may be a symptom of a medical condition. Thus, it may occur with other signs and symptoms of that condition. For example, if you have a cold, you may have a runny or stuffy nose. If you have gastroesophageal reflux disease, you may have a sour taste in your mouth.

A chronic cough can make you feel tired because you use a lot of energy to cough. It also can prevent you from sleeping well and interfere with work and socializing. A chronic cough also can cause headaches, chest pain, loss of bladder control, sweating, and, rarely, fractured ribs.

Sneezing And Allergy

Children are magnets for colds. But when the sniffles and sneezing won't go away for weeks, the culprit may be allergies.

Long-lasting sneezing, with a stuffy or runny nose, may signal the presence of allergic rhinitis—the collection of symptoms that affect the nose when you have an allergic reaction to something you breathe in and that lands on the lining inside the nose.

Allergies may be seasonal or can strike year-round (perennial). In most parts of the United States, plant pollens are often the cause of seasonal allergic rhinitis—more commonly called hay fever. Indoor substances, such as mold, dust mites, and pet dander, may cause the perennial kind.

Up to 40 percent of children suffer from allergic rhinitis. And children are more likely to develop allergies if one or both parents have allergies.

The U.S. Food and Drug Administration (FDA) regulates over-the-counter (OTC) and prescription medicines that offer allergy relief as well as allergen extracts used to diagnose and treat allergies.

(Sources: "Allergy Relief For Your Child," U.S. Department of Food and Drug Administration (FDA).)

How Is The Cause Of Cough Diagnosed?

Your doctor will diagnose the cause of your cough based on your medical history, a physical exam, and test results.

Medical History

Your doctor will likely ask questions about your cough. He or she may ask how long you've had it, whether you're coughing anything up (such as mucus, a slimy substance), and how much you cough.

Your doctor also may ask:

- About your medical history, including whether you have allergies, asthma, or other medical conditions.

- Whether you have heartburn or a sour taste in your mouth. These may be signs of gastroesophageal reflux disease (GERD).

- Whether you've recently had a cold or the flu.

- Whether you smoke or spend time around others who smoke.

- Whether you've been around air pollution, a lot of dust, or fumes.

Physical Exam

To check for signs of problems related to cough, your doctor will use a stethoscope to listen to your lungs. He or she will listen for wheezing (a whistling or squeaky sound when you breathe) or other abnormal sounds.

Diagnostic Tests

Your doctor may recommend tests based on the results of your medical history and physical exam. For example, if you have symptoms of GERD, your doctor may recommend a pH probe. This test measures the acid level of the fluid in your throat.

Other tests may include:

- **An exam of the mucus from your nose or throat.** This test can show whether you have a bacterial infection.

- **A chest X-ray.** A chest X-ray takes a picture of your heart and lungs. This test can help diagnose conditions such as pneumonia and lung cancer.

- **Lung function tests.** These tests measure how much air you can breathe in and out, how fast you can breathe air out, and how well your lungs deliver oxygen to your blood. Lung function tests can help diagnose asthma and other conditions.

- **An X-ray of the sinuses.** This test can help diagnose a sinus infection.

How Is Cough Treated?

The best way to treat a cough is to treat its cause. However, sometimes the cause is unknown. Other treatments, such as medicines and a vaporizer, can help relieve the cough itself.

Acute And Subacute Cough

An acute cough lasts less than 3 weeks. Common causes of an acute cough are a common cold or other upper respiratory infections. Examples of other upper respiratory infections include the flu, pneumonia, and whooping cough. An acute cough usually goes away after the illness that caused it is over. A subacute cough lasts 3 to 8 weeks. This type of cough remains even after a cold or other respiratory infection is over.

Studies show that antibiotics and cold medicines can't cure a cold. However, your doctor may prescribe medicines to treat another cause of an acute or subacute cough. For example, antibiotics may be given for pneumonia.

Chronic Cough

A chronic cough lasts more than 8 weeks. Common causes of a chronic cough are upper airway cough syndrome (UACS), asthma, and gastroesophageal reflux disease (GERD).

"UACS" is a term used to describe conditions that inflame the upper airways and cause a cough. Examples include sinus infections and allergies. These conditions can cause mucus (a slimy substance) to run down your throat from the back of your nose. This is called postnasal drip.

If you have a sinus infection, your doctor may prescribe antibiotics. He or she also may suggest you use a medicine that you spray into your nose. If allergies are causing your cough, your doctor may advise you to avoid the substances that you're allergic to (allergens) if possible.

If you have asthma, try to avoid irritants and allergens that make your asthma worse. Take your asthma medicines as your doctor prescribes.

GERD occurs if acid from your stomach backs up into your throat. Your doctor may prescribe a medicine to reduce acid in your stomach. You also may be able to relieve GERD symptoms by waiting 3 to 4 hours after a meal before lying down, and by sleeping with your head raised.

Smoking also can cause a chronic cough. If you smoke, it's important to quit. Talk with your doctor about programs and products that can help you quit smoking. Also, try to avoid secondhand smoke. Many hospitals have programs that help people quit smoking, or hospital staff can refer you to a program.

Other causes of a chronic cough include respiratory infections, chronic bronchitis, bronchiectasis, lung cancer, and heart failure. Treatments for these causes may include medicines, procedures, and other therapies. Treatment also may include avoiding irritants and allergens and quitting smoking.

If your chronic cough is due to a medicine you're taking, your doctor may prescribe a different medicine.

Cough In Children

No evidence shows that cough and cold medicines help children recover more quickly from colds. These medicines can even harm children.

Living With Cough

If you have a cough, you can take steps to recover from the condition that's causing the cough. You also can take steps to relieve your cough. Ongoing care and lifestyle changes can help you.

Treating The Cough Rather Than The Cause

Coughing is important because it helps clear your airways of irritants, such as smoke and mucus (a slimy substance). Coughing also helps prevent infections.

Cough medicines usually are used only when the cause of the cough is unknown and the cough causes a lot of discomfort.

Medicines can help control a cough and make it easier to cough up mucus. Your doctor may recommend medicines such as:

- **Prescription cough suppressants, also called antitussives.** These medicines can help relieve a cough. However, they're usually used when nothing else works. No evidence shows that over-the-counter (OTC) cough suppressants relieve a cough.
- **Expectorants.** These medicines may loosen mucus, making it easier to cough up.
- **Bronchodilators.** These medicines relax your airways.

Other treatments also may relieve an irritated throat and loosen mucus. Examples include using a cool-mist humidifier or steam vaporizer and drinking enough fluids. Examples of fluids are water, soup, and juice. Ask your doctor how much fluid you need.

Ongoing Care

Follow the treatment plan your doctor gives you for treating the cause of your cough. Take all medicines as your doctor prescribes. If you're using antibiotics, continue to take the medicine until it's all gone. You may start to feel better before you finish the medicine, but you should continue to take it.

Ask your doctor about ways to relieve your cough. He or she may recommend cough medicines. These medicines usually are used only when the cause of a cough is unknown and the cough is causing a lot of discomfort.

A cool-mist humidifier or steam vaporizer may help relieve an irritated throat and loosen mucus. Getting enough fluids (for example, water, soup, or juice) may have the same effect. Ask your doctor about how much fluid you need.

Your doctor will let you know when to schedule follow-up care.

Lifestyle Changes

If you smoke, quit. Ask your doctor about programs and products that can help you quit smoking.

Try to avoid irritants and allergens that make you cough. Examples of irritants include cigarette smoke, air pollution, paint fumes, and scented products like perfumes or air fresheners. Examples of allergens include dust, animal dander, mold, and pollens from trees, grasses, and flowers.

Follow a healthy diet and be as physically active as you can. A healthy diet includes a variety of fruits, vegetables, and whole grains. It also includes lean meats, poultry, fish, and fat-free or low-fat milk or milk products. A healthy diet also is low in saturated fat, trans fat, cholesterol, sodium (salt), and added sugar.

Chapter 13

Allergic Rhinitis

What Is Allergic Rhinitis?[1]

People with seasonal allergies (also called hay fever or allergic rhinitis) react to pollen from plants. Symptoms may include sneezing, coughing, a runny or stuffy nose, and itching in the eyes, nose, mouth, and throat. If you have an allergy, your immune system reacts to something that doesn't bother most other people.

Patients with allergic rhinitis may have both nasal and non-nasal symptoms. The main nasal symptoms of allergic rhinitis are nasal itching (i.e., nasal pruritus), sneezing, rhinorrhea, and nasal congestion. Nasal pruritus and sneezing are induced by sensory nerve stimulation, whereas congestion results from vasodilation with resultant engorgement of cavernous sinusoids. Rhinorrhea can be induced by increased vascular permeability, as well as direct glandular secretion. Important non-nasal symptoms commonly associated with allergic rhinitis include eye itching, tearing, eye redness, and itching of ears and/or palate.

(Source: "Allergic Rhinitis: Developing Drug Products For Treatment Guidance For Industry," U.S. Food and Drug Administration (FDA).)

About This Chapter: This chapter includes text excerpted from documents published by two public domain sources. Text under the headings marked 1 are excerpted from "Seasonal Allergies At A Glance," National Center for Complementary and Integrative Health (NCCIH), September 24, 2017; Text under the headings marked 2 are excerpted from "Allergies," U.S. Department of Food and Drug Administration (FDA), December 3, 2014. Reviewed November 2017.

Symptoms Of Hay Fever[2]

- Sneezing
- Runny or clogged nose
- Coughing
- Itchy eyes, nose, and throat
- Watery eyes
- Red, swollen eyes

Why Do Some People Have Allergies And Hay Fever?[2]

No one is sure what causes allergies. You are more likely to have hay fever if your parents have it.

What Kinds Of Tests Check For Allergies?[2]

- Skin tests—Your doctor may also use a needle to put a small amount of allergen into your skin. After a few minutes, the reaction tells your doctor if you have allergies.
- Blood tests—Your doctor may use a blood test to look for a protein in your blood called IgE. This protein is made by people with allergies and hay fever. It also helps fight certain types of infection.

Both tests look for certain disease-fighting cells (antibodies). Your body makes these cells to match whatever it is fighting. Your antibodies tell doctors what you are allergic to.

How Are Allergies And Hay Fever Treated?[2]

Your doctor can help you decide what to do. You can:

- Avoid the things that cause your symptoms.
- Use medicines.
- Get allergy shots.

Allergy shots contain small amounts of what you are allergic to. At first, shots may be given every week to lessen your symptoms. The shots are usually continued for 3 to 5 years.

Hay Fever Versus Colds[2]

Table 13.1. Hay Fever Versus Colds

	Hay Fever	Colds
Signs	Signs can include running or stuffed nose, sneezing, wheezing, itchy, and watery eyes.	Signs can include fever, aches and pains stuffed nose, sneezing, and watery eyes.
Warning Time	Symptoms begin right away.	Symptoms usually take a few days to start.
Duration	Symptoms last as long as you are around the allergen.	Symptoms should clear up within a week.

Complementary Health Approaches For Allergic Rhinitis[1]

Many complementary health approaches have been studied for allergic rhinitis. There's some evidence that a few may be helpful.

Mind And Body Practices

- A 2015 evaluation of 13 studies of acupuncture for allergic rhinitis, involving a total of 2,365 participants, found evidence that this approach may be helpful.

- Rinsing the sinuses with a neti pot (a device that comes from the Ayurvedic tradition) or with other devices, such as nebulizers or spray, pump, or squirt bottles, may be a useful addition to conventional treatment for allergic rhinitis.

Natural Products

- An evaluation of six studies of the herb butterbur for allergic rhinitis, involving a total of 720 participants, indicated that butterbur may be helpful.

- Researchers have been investigating probiotics (live microorganisms that may have health benefits) for diseases of the immune system, including allergies. Although some studies have had promising results, the overall evidence on probiotics and allergic rhinitis is inconsistent. It's possible that some types of probiotics might be helpful but that others are not.

- It's been thought that eating honey might help to relieve pollen allergies because honey contains small amounts of pollen and might help people build up a tolerance to it.

Another possibility is that honey could act as an antihistamine or anti-inflammatory agent. Only a few studies have examined the effects of honey in people with seasonal allergies, and their results have been inconsistent.

- Many other natural products have been studied for allergic rhinitis, including astragalus, capsaicin, grape seed extract, omega-3 fatty acids, Pycnogenol (French maritime pine bark extract), quercetin, spirulina, stinging nettle, and an herb used in Ayurvedic medicine called tinospora or guduchi. In all instances, the evidence is either inconsistent or too limited to show whether these products are helpful.

Side Effects And Risks[1]

- People can get infections if they use neti pots or other nasal rinsing devices improperly. The U.S. Food and Drug Administration (FDA) has information on how to rinse your sinuses safely.

  - Most important is the source of water that is used with nasal rinsing devices. According to the FDA, tap water that is not filtered, treated, or processed in specific ways is not safe for use as a nasal rinse. Sterile water is safe; over-the-counter (OTC) nasal rinsing products that contain sterile saline (salt water) are available.

  - Some tap water contains low levels of organisms, such as bacteria and protozoa, including amoebas, which may be safe to swallow because stomach acid kills them. But these organisms can stay alive in nasal passages and cause potentially serious infections. Improper use of neti pots may have caused two deaths in 2011 in Louisiana from a rare brain infection that the state health department linked to tap water contaminated with an amoeba called Naegleria fowleri.

- Acupuncture is generally considered safe when performed by an experienced practitioner using sterile needles. Improperly performed acupuncture can cause potentially serious side effects.

- Raw butterbur extracts contain pyrrolizidine alkaloids, which can cause liver damage and cancer. Extracts of butterbur that are almost completely free from these alkaloids are available. However, no studies have proven that the long-term use of butterbur products, including the reduced-alkaloid products, is safe.

- In healthy people, probiotics usually have only minor side effects, if any. However, in people with underlying health problems (for example, weakened immune systems), serious complications such as infections have occasionally been reported.

- Be cautious about using herbs or bee products for any purpose. Some herbs, such as chamomile and echinacea, may cause allergic reactions in people who are allergic to related plants. Also, people with pollen allergies may have allergic reactions to bee products, such as bee pollen, honey, royal jelly, and propolis (a hive sealant made by bees from plant resins). Children under 1 year of age should not eat honey.

- Talk to your healthcare provider about the best way to manage your seasonal allergies, especially if you're considering or using a dietary supplement. Be aware that some supplements may interact with medications or other supplements or have side effects of their own. Keep in mind that most dietary supplements have not been tested in pregnant women, nursing mothers, or children.

Chapter 14

Sinusitis

A sinus infection (sinusitis) does not typically need to be treated with antibiotics in order to get better. If you or your child is diagnosed with a sinus infection, your healthcare professional can decide if antibiotics are needed.

Signs And Symptoms

Common signs and symptoms of a sinus infection include:

- Headache

- Stuffy or runny nose

- Loss of the sense of smell

- Facial pain or pressure

- Postnasal drip (mucus drips down the throat from the nose)

- Sore throat

- Fever

- Coughing

- Fatigue (being tired)

- Bad breath

About This Chapter: This chapter includes text excerpted from "Sinus Infection (Sinusitis)," Centers for Disease Control and Prevention (CDC), September 25, 2017.

Symptom Relief

Rest, over-the-counter (OTC) medicines and other self-care methods may help you to feel better. Always use over-the-counter products as directed since many over-the-counter products are not recommended for children of certain ages.

Causes

Sinus infections occur when fluid is trapped or blocked in the sinuses, allowing germs to grow. Sinus infections are usually (9 out of 10 cases in adults; 5–7 out of 10 cases in children) caused by a virus. They are less commonly (1 out of 10 cases in adults; 3–5 out of 10 cases in children) caused by bacteria.

Other conditions can cause symptoms similar to a sinus infection, including:

- Allergies

- Pollutants (airborne chemicals or irritants)

- Fungal infections

Risk Factors

Several conditions can increase your risk of getting a sinus infection:

- A previous respiratory tract infection, such as the common cold

- Structural problems within the sinuses

- A weak immune system or taking drugs that weaken the immune system

- Nasal polyps

- Allergies

In children, the following are also risk factors for a sinus infection:

- Going to daycare
- Using a pacifier
- Drinking a bottle while laying down
- Being exposed to secondhand smoke

When To Seek Medical Care

See a healthcare professional if you or your child has any of the following:

- Temperature higher than 100.4°F

- Symptoms that are getting worse or lasting more than 10 days

- Multiple sinus infections in the past year

- Symptoms that are not relieved with over-the-counter medicines

If your child is younger than three months of age and has a fever, it's important to call your healthcare professional right away.

You may have chronic sinusitis if your sinus infection lasts more than 8 weeks or if you have more than 4 sinus infections each year. If you are diagnosed with chronic sinusitis, or believe you may have chronic sinusitis, you should visit your healthcare professional for evaluation. Chronic sinusitis can be caused by nasal growths, allergies, or respiratory tract infections (viral, bacterial, or fungal).

Diagnosis And Treatment

Your healthcare professional will determine if you or your child has a sinus infection by asking about symptoms and doing a physical examination. Sometimes they will also swab the inside of your nose.

Antibiotics may be needed if the sinus infection is likely to be caused by bacteria. Antibiotics will not help a sinus infection caused by a virus or an irritation in the air (like secondhand smoke). These infections will almost always get better on their own. Antibiotic treatment in these cases may even cause harm in both children and adults.

If symptoms continue for more than 10 days, schedule a follow-up appointment with your healthcare professional for re-evaluation.

Prevention

There are several steps you can take to help prevent a sinus infection, including:

- Practice good hand hygiene

- Keep you and your child up to date with recommended immunizations

- Avoid close contact with people who have colds or other upper respiratory infections

- Avoid smoking and exposure to secondhand smoke

- Use a clean humidifier to moisten the air at home

Chapter 15

Asthma And Allergies

Asthma is a chronic disease that affects your airways. Your airways are tubes that carry air in and out of your lungs. If you have asthma, the inside walls of your airways become sore and swollen. That makes them very sensitive, and they may react strongly to things that you are allergic to or find irritating.

If someone in your family has allergies or asthma, make your home a healthier place by getting rid of the things that can cause allergy symptoms or an asthma attack.

What Can Cause Allergy Symptoms Or An Asthma Attack?

Things that can cause allergy symptoms are called allergens. Asthma attacks can be caused by irritants (things that can irritate the lungs) or allergens. Different people will react to different allergens and irritants.

Common causes of allergy symptoms and asthma attacks at home include:

- Mold or dampness

- Dust mites (tiny bugs that live in beds and carpets)

- Pets with fur, including cats and dogs

About This Chapter: This chapter includes text excerpted from "Prevent Allergies And Asthma Attacks At Home," Office of Disease Prevention and Health Promotion (ODPHP), U.S. Department of Health and Human Services (HHS), May 15, 2017.

- Cockroaches (roaches and their droppings may cause asthma)

- Mice, rats, and other rodents

- Secondhand smoke

- Wood smoke

- Strong fragrances

Take Action!

Follow these steps to make your home a healthier place for people with allergies or asthma.

Find out what causes your allergy symptoms or asthma attacks.

If you or someone in your family has asthma, it's important to figure out what can trigger (cause) an asthma attack. Asthma triggers can be different for different people.

Ask your doctor about getting an allergy test. This test can help you know what exactly is causing your allergies.

When you know what you are allergic to—or what your asthma triggers are—you can take steps to get rid of or avoid those things in your home.

Keep allergens and irritants out of the bedroom.

- Cover your mattresses and pillows in "dust proof" (or "allergen proof") covers.

- Wash all your bedding in very hot water (at least 130°F) once a week. Go to a laundromat if the water in your home doesn't get that hot.

- Keep stuffed animals off the bed.

- If you have pets that you are allergic to (like cats or dogs), keep them out of the bedroom.

- If possible, remove all carpets. It's easier to keep bare floors clean.

Control moisture to prevent mold.

Keep your home dry to prevent mold. Mold can start to grow in wet or damp places within just 1 or 2 days.

- If you have a water leak, clean up the water right away. Fix the leak as soon as possible.

- When you take a shower, run the bathroom fan or open the window for at least 20 minutes afterward.

- Check the humidity level in your home with a moisture or humidity meter (available at a hardware store).

- Use a dehumidifier or air conditioner to keep the humidity level in your home below 60 percent. A humidity level between 30 and 50 percent is best.

If you rent your home and there's mold in it, you may be able to ask your landlord or property manager to clean up the mold.

What Health Effects Are Linked To Air Pollution?

Over the past 30 years, researchers have unearthed a wide array of health effects which are believed to be associated with air pollution exposure. Among them are respiratory diseases (including asthma and changes in lung function), cardiovascular diseases, adverse pregnancy outcomes (such as preterm birth), and even death.

What If The Air In My Home Is Too Dry?

While moist (wet) air can lead to mold, dry air can be uncomfortable. If the air in your home is dry in the winter, you can use a humidifier. Just be sure to still keep the humidity level between 30 and 50 percent.

Keep pests out of your home.

Rodents (mice and rats) and cockroaches can trigger allergy or asthma attacks if you are allergic to them. Take these steps to help prevent pests:

- Fix leaks in sinks and toilets.
- Put trays under your plants, radiators, and refrigerator. Check the trays for water and clean them often.
- Store food (including pet food) in closed containers.
- Clean up crumbs and spills right away.
- Fill in cracks or holes that could be good indoor hiding places for pests.
- Put screens in your windows and doors.
- If you see roaches or rodents, call a pest control company.

Make a no-smoking rule in your home.

Cigarette smoke, including secondhand smoke, can make asthma worse. And babies who live in homes where people smoke are at higher risk of developing asthma.

If you have guests who smoke, ask them to smoke outside. If you smoke, make a plan to quit today.

Avoid burning wood inside your home.

Breathing too much smoke from a wood-burning stove or fireplace can cause an asthma attack. If you can avoid it, don't burn wood in your home.

Chapter 16

Hypersensitivity Pneumonitis

Hypersensitivity pneumonitis is a rare immune system disorder that affects the lungs. It occurs in some people after they breathe in certain substances they encounter in the environment. These substances trigger their immune systems, causing short- or long-term inflammation, especially in a part of the lungs called the interstitium. This inflammation makes it harder for the lungs to function properly and may even permanently damage the lungs. If diagnosed, some types of hypersensitivity pneumonitis are treatable by avoiding exposure to the environmental substances or with medicines such as corticosteroids that reduce inflammation. If the condition goes untreated or is not well controlled over time, the chronic inflammation can cause irreversible scarring of the lungs that may severely impair their ability to function.

Other Names
Extrinsic allergic alveolitis, bird fancier's lung, farmer's lung, hot tub lung, and humidifier lung.

Causes

Hypersensitivity pneumonitis is caused by repeated exposure to environmental substances that cause inflammation in the lungs when inhaled. These substances include certain:

- Bacteria and mycobacteria

- Fungi or molds

About This Chapter: This chapter includes text excerpted from "Hypersensitivity Pneumonitis," National Heart, Lung, and Blood Institute (NHLBI), May 27, 2016.

- Proteins

- Chemicals

Where Can These Substances Be Found In The Environment?

Common environmental sources of substances that can cause hypersensitivity pneumonitis are:

- Animal furs

- Air conditioner, humidifier, and ventilation systems

- Bird droppings and feathers

- Contaminated foods such as cheese, grapes, barley, sugarcane

- Contaminated industry products or materials such as sausage casings and corks

- Contaminated metalworking fluid

- Hardwood dusts

- Hay or grain animal feed

- Hot tubs

Because this condition is caused by different substances found in many environmental sources, doctors once thought they were treating different lung diseases. Research also revealed that the hypersensitivity pneumonitis is triggered by different causative substances.

Why Does Hypersensitivity Pneumonitis Only Occur In Some People?

If you have hypersensitivity pneumonitis, your body's immune system reacts strongly to certain substances. Differences in our immune systems may explain why some people have strong reactions after breathing in certain substances, while others who breathe those same substances do not.

Tell Me More

Normally, the immune system in the lungs monitors inhaled substances. The immune system is activated when it recognizes a portion of the substance called the antigen as foreign. The activated immune system produces molecules that cause normal levels of inflammation, such as increased levels of immune cells and factors including antibodies that recognize and help clear the foreign substance. Normally after clearing the substance, the immune system shuts off and the inflammation stops. Usually, these processes are well controlled.

The immune systems of people with hypersensitivity pneumonitis are unable to shut down these normal inflammation processes, especially in the lung interstitium. The interstitium is a space where the lung's air sacs, called alveoli, come in contact with blood vessels and a small amount of connective tissue. When there is high level of inflammation in the lungs, immune cells begin to collect in this space. These uncontrolled levels of inflammation in the lungs cause the signs, symptoms, and complications of this condition.

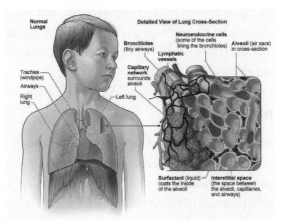

Figure 16.1. Lymphatic Vessel

In the lung interstitium, alveoli air sacs come into contact with the blood vessels and connective tissues of the lung. If you have hypersensitivity pneumonitis, your body's immune system reacts strongly to certain inhaled substances, causing inflammation especially in the interstitium or interstitial space.

Risk Factors

Certain factors affect your risk of developing hypersensitivity pneumonitis. These factors include age, environment or occupation, family history and genetics, lifestyle habits, other medical conditions, and sex or gender.

Age

Although hypersensitivity pneumonitis can occur at any age, people tend to be diagnosed with this condition between 50 and 55 years of age. Hypersensitivity pneumonitis is a common type of chronic interstitial lung disease in children.

Environment Or Occupation

Repeated exposure to certain substances that cause the condition, possibly while working in occupations where environmental sources are common, can increase your risk of developing hypersensitivity pneumonitis. Certain occupations—such as farmers or people who breed animals or birds, cheese washers, woodworkers, and wine makers—have a greater chance of exposure to causative substances. However, you may be exposed to environmental sources in your home or elsewhere. Even having pets such as birds in the home can increase your risk of hypersensitivity pneumonitis.

Alone, environmental exposure to causative substances is not enough to cause hypersensitivity pneumonitis. An estimated 85 to 95 percent of people exposed to causative substances either never develop hypersensitivity pneumonitis or they experience a mild immune reaction with no obvious signs or symptoms or disease.

Family History And Genetics

Genetics is thought to predispose some people to have strong immune responses and develop hypersensitivity pneumonitis after repeat exposures to a causative substance. In some populations, family history of pulmonary fibrosis or hypersensitivity pneumonitis may increase the risk of developing hypersensitivity pneumonitis. When hypersensitivity pneumonitis occurs in relatives it is called familial hypersensitivity pneumonitis.

Researchers are beginning to map genetic variations in immune system proteins that may increase the risk for developing hypersensitivity pneumonitis. These differences may explain why immune cells respond differently between people who do or do not develop hypersensitivity pneumonitis after the same exposure to a causative substance.

Lifestyle Habits

Smoking is not thought to increase the risk of developing hypersensitivity pneumonitis. However, smoking can worsen chronic hypersensitivity pneumonitis and cause complications. If you have hypersensitivity pneumonitis, learn why doctors recommend quitting smoking.

Other Medical Conditions

Some viral infections later in life may increase the risk of developing hypersensitivity pneumonitis.

Sex Or Gender

Men and women can have hypersensitivity pneumonitis. Some small studies found this condition to be slightly more common in women.

Currently, there are no screening methods to determine who will or will not develop hypersensitivity pneumonitis. you avoid common environmental sources of substances known to cause this condition. If you are at risk for hypersensitivity pneumonitis, your doctor may recommend you avoid common environmental sources of substances known to cause this condition.

Signs, Symptoms, And Complications

Signs and symptoms vary between acute, subacute, and chronic types of hypersensitivity pneumonitis. If your condition is not diagnosed or well controlled by treatment, it can lead to irreversible lung damage and other potentially fatal complications.

Signs And Symptoms

The following are common signs and symptoms of acute, subacute, and chronic hypersensitivity pneumonitis.

Type of Hypersensitivity Pneumonitis	Signs and Symptoms								
	Flu-like Illness (fever, chills, muscle or joint pain, headache)	Rales	Cough	Chronic Bronchitis	Shortness of Breath	Anorexia or Weight Loss	Fatigue	Lung Fibrosis	Clubbing of Fingers or Toes
Acute	✓	✓	✓						
Subacute		✓	✓	✓	✓	✓			
Chronic			✓	✓	✓	✓	✓	✓	✓

Figure 16.2. Signs And Symptoms Of Acute, Subacute, And Chronic Hypersensitivity Pneumonitis

Signs and symptoms of acute, subacute, and chronic hypersensitivity pneumonitis may include flu-like illness including fever, chills, muscle or joint pain, or headaches; rales; cough; chronic bronchitis; shortness of breath; anorexia or weight loss; fatigue; fibrosis of the lungs; and clubbing of fingers or toes.

While some signs and symptoms occur in several types of hypersensitivity pneumonitis, they may vary in severity. The exact signs and symptoms you experience also may vary.

Tell Me More

Acute hypersensitivity pneumonitis is the most common form of this condition. It is thought to occur as a result of a short period of exposure to a large amount of causative substance. Symptoms usually occur within 9 hours of being exposed again to a substance that triggers your immune system. If an additional exposure does not occur, symptoms usually resolve after a few days. Subacute and chronic forms of hypersensitivity pneumonitis occur after multiple or continuous exposures to small amounts of causative substance. Approximately 5 percent of patients develop chronic disease.

Complications

Hypersensitivity pneumonitis may cause the following potentially fatal complications if the condition is not diagnosed or well controlled by treatment.

- **Irreversible lung damage and permanently reduced lung function** because of severe fibrosis and impaired ability to oxygenate the blood during normal breathing.

- **Pulmonary hypertension** due to damage of blood vessels in the lungs.

- **Heart failure** because inflammation makes it harder for the heart to pump blood to and through the lungs.

Diagnosis

To diagnose hypersensitivity pneumonitis, your doctor will collect your medical history to understand your symptoms and see if you have an exposure history to possible causative substances. Your doctor will perform a physical exam and may order diagnostic tests and procedures. Based on this information, your doctor may able to determine whether you have acute, subacute, or chronic hypersensitivity pneumonitis.

Diagnostic Tests And Procedures

To diagnose hypersensitivity pneumonitis, your doctor may order:

- **Blood tests** to detect high levels of white blood cells and other immune cells and factors in your blood that indicate your immune system is activated and causing inflammation somewhere in your body.

- **Bronchoalveolar lavage (BAL)** to collect fluid from your lungs that can be tested for high levels of white blood cells and other immune cells. High levels of these cells mean your body is making an immune response in your lungs, but low levels do not rule out hypersensitivity pneumonitis.

- **Computed tomography (CT) scan** to image the lungs and look for inflammation or damage such as fibrosis. CT scans, particularly high-resolution ones, can help distinguish between types of hypersensitivity pneumonitis.

- **Inhalation challenge tests** to see if a controlled exposure to a suspected causative substance triggers your immune system and the onset of common signs and symptoms such as an increase in temperature, increase in white blood cell levels, rales that are heard during a physical exam, or reduced lung function. A positive test can confirm an inhaled substance triggers your immune system. A negative test does not rule out that you have hypersensitivity pneumonitis, because it may mean a different untested environmental substance is causing your condition. Before having this test, talk to your doctor about the benefits and possible risks of this procedure.

- **Lung biopsies** to see if your lung tissue shows signs of inflammation, fibrosis, or other changes known to occur in hypersensitivity pneumonitis.

- **Lung function tests** to see if you show signs of restriction such as reduced breathing capacity or abnormal blood oxygen levels and check if you have obstructed airways. These tests help assess the severity of your lung disease and when repeated they can help monitor whether your condition is stable or worsening over time. Lung function tests may be normal between acute flares.

- **Precipitin tests** to see if you have antibodies in your blood that recognize and bind to a causative substance. While a positive test means that you have been exposed to a substance, it cannot confirm you have hypersensitivity pneumonitis. This is because some people without this condition also have antibodies in their blood to these substances. If you have antibodies to a substance, your doctor may have you perform an inhalation challenge test to see if a new exposure to the same substance can activate your immune system and cause a new acute flare.

- **Chest X-rays** to image the lungs and look for inflammation or damage such as fibrosis in your lungs.

Tell Me More

Chest X-ray and CT scans, lung biopsies, and lung function tests may help your doctor diagnose the type of hypersensitivity pneumonitis that you have.

- **Chest X-rays and CT scans** may show little to no inflammation in your lungs during the early phase of acute disease, but they will show obvious signs of inflammation and tissue damage such as fibrosis in subacute and chronic hypersensitivity pneumonitis.

- **Lung function tests** may detect breathing difficulties, small airflow blockages, or reduced lung function in acute hypersensitivity pneumonitis. These problems may worsen and progress to severe lung restriction in subacute and chronic hypersensitivity pneumonitis.

- **Lung biopsies** will reveal inflammation, fibrosis, and possibly granulomas in subacute and chronic hypersensitivity pneumonitis. They are not usually performed for acute hypersensitivity pneumonitis.

Your medical and exposure histories can help your doctor diagnose acute hypersensitivity pneumonitis and possibly identify the substance causing your condition. This is because the exposure will have occurred right before your acute symptoms started.

Is It Hard To Diagnose This Condition?

It can take months or even years for your doctor to diagnose hypersensitivity pneumonitis in you or your child. Learn why hypersensitivity pneumonitis can be hard to diagnose.

- **There are no clear exposure histories to potential causative substances before having symptoms.** This occurs in up to 50 percent of patients who are later diagnosed with hypersensitivity pneumonitis. Despite hypersensitivity pneumonitis being a common childhood interstitial lung disease, children are often diagnosed late after the condition has progressed to chronic disease. This is because children tend to be exposed to small amounts of causative substance over long periods of time, which does not trigger obvious acute symptoms and makes it very difficult to determine their exposure history.

- **Other conditions may cause similar signs and symptoms.** Before diagnosing hypersensitivity pneumonitis, your doctor must rule out: unintentional effects of medicines such as bleomycin, methotrexate, or nitrofurantoin; lung infections such as pneumonia or the flu (influenza); smoking-related lung disease; connective tissue disease; bleeding in the lungs; idiopathic pulmonary fibrosis; sarcoidosis; and lung cancer.

- **Diagnostic features seen in chest X-rays, CT scans, and lung biopsies may differ between children and adults.** Even when a person's exposure history is known or hypersensitivity pneumonitis is suspected, doctors look for diagnostic features in chest X-rays, CT scans, and lung biopsies that are indicators of the disease in adults. More research is needed to help map diagnostic features for children with this condition.

Treatment

Treatments for hypersensitivity pneumonitis usually include avoidance strategies and medicines. Occasionally, lung transplants are used to treat severe chronic disease in some patients.

Avoidance Strategies

If your doctor is able to identify the environmental substance that causes your hypersensitivity pneumonitis, he or she will recommend that you adopt the following avoidance strategies.

- **Remove** the causative substance if possible

- **Replace** workplace or other products with available alternatives that do not contain the substance responsible for your condition

- **Alter** work processes so you don't continue to breathe in the causative substance

- **Stay away** from known sources of your causative substance

Medicines

If avoidance strategies do not work for your condition, your doctor may prescribe corticosteroids or other immunosuppressive medicines to treat your condition. The choice, dose, and duration of these medicines will depend on your condition and medical history. Acute and subacute types of hypersensitivity pneumonitis usually respond well to these treatments.

Depending on your condition, your doctor also may prescribe some of the following supportive therapies.

- **Oxygen therapy** as needed for low levels of oxygen in the blood.
- **Bronchodilators** to relax the muscles in the airways and open your airways to make breathing easier.
- **Opioids** to control shortness of breath or chronic cough that is resistant to other treatments. Regular (e.g., several times a day, for several weeks or more) or longer use of opioids can lead to physical dependence and possibly addiction.

Lung Transplants

If your condition is not adequately controlled by avoidance strategies or medicines and you develop serious complications, you may be a candidate for a lung transplant. During this procedure, healthy donor lung will be transplanted into you to replace the damaged lung. Two important things to know:

- **This procedure is not a cure.** This is because your immune system will be the same after the procedure. This means that if you are exposed again to the substances that triggers your immune system, new inflammation may damage the transplanted donor lung tissue.

- **This procedure is not for everyone.** Even if you are a candidate for this procedure, it may be difficult to find a matching organ donor. Lung transplants are serious medical procedures with their own risks. Talk to your doctor about what procedures are right for you.

Tell Me More

Treatment is more successful when hypersensitivity pneumonitis is diagnosed in the early stages of the disease, before permanent irreversible lung damage has occurred. As new data emerges, doctors are becoming more aware of the unique treatment needs for children with hypersensitivity pneumonitis.

Living With

If you have hypersensitivity pneumonitis, you can take steps to control the condition and prevent complications by receiving routine follow-up care, monitoring your condition, preventing new acute flares and complications, and learning about and preparing for serious complications.

Receive Routine Follow-Up Care

In addition to treatments you are using to control your condition, your doctor may recommend other medical care to improve your quality of life, vaccines to prevent lung infections, and lifestyle changes such as physical activity and quitting smoking to improve overall health and avoid some complications.

- **Other medical care:** Your doctor may evaluate how your condition is affecting your activity level and mental health. To improve your quality of life, your doctor may recommend other treatments to address pain, fatigue, or mental health concerns that you may have.

- **Vaccines:** Remember that your condition causes you to have reduced lung function, particularly if you have subacute or chronic hypersensitivity pneumonitis. Your doctor may recommend that you receive routine pneumococcal and flu (influenza) vaccines to avoid lung infections that can further impair your reduced lung function.

- **Physical activity:** Patients with hypersensitivity pneumonitis benefit from regular exercise. Before starting any exercise program, ask your doctor about what level of physical activity is right for you.

- **Quitting smoking:** If you smoke, quit. Although smoking does not increase the risk of developing hypersensitivity pneumonitis, some studies suggest smoking can worsen disease and shorten survival for people with chronic hypersensitivity pneumonitis compared to nonsmokers with chronic hypersensitivity pneumonitis. Another study reported lung cancer in patients who smoked and had chronic hypersensitivity pneumonitis.

Monitor Your Condition

If you have been diagnosed with subacute or chronic hypersensitivity pneumonitis, your doctor may recommend follow-up testing to see how well your treatment is working and if your disease is improving, stable, or worse. To monitor your condition, your doctor may recommend repeating tests used earlier to diagnose hypersensitivity pneumonitis such as chest X-rays, computed tomography (CT) scans, or lung function tests.

Your doctor may determine your disease is worse if you have new or more severe fibrosis or lung function problems. High-resolution CT scans may be more informative than lung function tests at assessing disease progression.

There is a growing recognition that disease tends to be worse, such as greater lung fibrosis, if it starts in childhood or early adult life. Therefore, more careful monitoring may be required for younger patients with hypersensitivity pneumonitis.

Prevent New Acute Flares And Serious Complications Over Your Lifetime

To help prevent new acute flares and complications, your doctor may recommend tests to identify the substances causing your condition, as well as additional screening tests to prevent potentially fatal complications.

- **Identification of substances causing your condition:** If you do not know the environmental substances causing your condition, your doctor may recommend diagnostic precipitin and inhalation challenge tests. Identification can help avoid the environmental sources of the substances causing your condition. Successful avoidance strategies can help you live a longer, prevent new acute flares, and slow or stop progression to chronic disease with serious complications.

- **Screening for serious complications:** If you have been diagnosed with chronic hypersensitivity pneumonitis, your doctor may recommend echocardiography and right-heart catheterization to evaluate pulmonary artery pressure and screen for pulmonary hypertension. Pulmonary hypertension can occur in people who have chronic hypersensitivity pneumonitis, particularly in patients with more severe disease who have poorer lung function and reduced exercise capacity

Learn The Warning Signs Of Serious Complications And Have A Plan

Always notify your doctor if your symptoms suddenly worsen. Your doctor will need to rule out other causes including infection and order repeat chest imaging tests. If these chest imaging tests show new findings without evidence of another cause, your doctor may modify your hypersensitivity pneumonitis treatment plan to better control your condition. Talk to your doctor and agree on a clinical decision plan to help you know when to seek urgent medical care.

Chapter 17

Eye Allergies

> Pink, itchy eyes? Pink eye—or conjunctivitis—is common and spreads easily. It sometimes needs medical treatment, depending on the cause. Know the symptoms, when to seek treatment, and how to help prevent it.

Pink Eye

Pink eye, also known as conjunctivitis, is one of the most common and treatable eye conditions in the world in both children and adults. It is an inflammation of the conjunctiva, the thin, clear tissue that lines the inside of the eyelid and the white part of the eyeball. This inflammation makes blood vessels more visible and gives the eye a pink or reddish color.

What Causes Pink Eye?

There are four main causes of pink eye:

• Viruses

• Bacteria

• Allergens (like pet dander or dust mites)

About This Chapter: Text under the heading "Pink Eye" is excerpted from "Pink Eye: Usually Mild And Easy To Treat," Centers for Disease Control and Prevention (CDC), March 20, 2017; Text under the heading "Vernal Keratoconjunctivitis" is excerpted from "Vernal Keratoconjunctivitis," Genetic and Rare Diseases Information Center (GARD), National Center for Advancing Translational Sciences (NCATS), December 7, 2011. Reviewed November 2017.

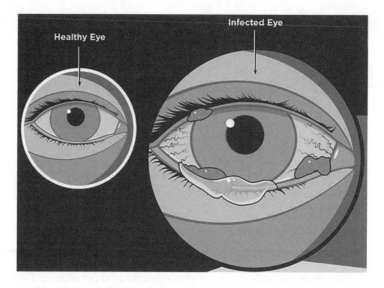

Figure 17.1. Healthy Versus Infected Eye

(Source: "Help Protect Yourself From Getting And Spreading Pink Eye (Conjunctivitis)," Centers for Disease Control and Prevention (CDC).)

- Irritants (like smog or swimming pool chlorine) that infect or irritate the eye and eyelid lining

It can be difficult to determine the exact cause of pink eye because some signs and symptoms may be the same no matter the cause.

What Are The Symptoms Of Pink Eye?

The symptoms of pink eye may vary depending on the cause but usually include:

- Redness or swelling of the white of the eye or inside the eyelids

- Increased amount of tears

- Eye discharge which may be clear, yellow, white or green

- Itchy, irritated, and/or burning eyes

- Increased sensitivity to light

- Gritty feeling in the eye

- Crusting of the eyelids or lashes

When To See A Healthcare Provider?

Most cases of pink eye are mild and get better on their own, even without treatment. However, there are times when it is important to see a healthcare provider for specific treatment and/or follow-up. You should see a healthcare provider if you have pink eye along with any of the following:

- Moderate to severe pain in your eye(s)

- Sensitivity to light or blurred vision

- Intense redness in the eye(s)

- A weakened immune system, for example from HIV or cancer treatment

- Symptoms that get worse or don't improve, including bacterial pink eye that does not improve after 24 hours of antibiotic use

- Pre-existing eye conditions that may put you at risk for complications or severe infection

How Do I Stop Pink Eye From Spreading?

Pink eye caused by a virus or bacteria is very contagious and spreads easily and quickly from person to person. Pink eye that is caused by allergens or irritants is not contagious, but it is possible to develop a secondary infection caused by a virus or bacteria that is contagious. You can reduce the risk of getting or spreading pink eye by following some simple self-care steps:

- Wash your hands

- Avoid touching or rubbing your eyes

- Avoid sharing makeup, contact lenses and containers, and eyeglasses

Pink Eye In Newborns

A newborn baby who has symptoms of pink eye should see a healthcare provider. Pink eye in newborns can be caused by an infection, irritation, or a blocked tear duct.

Neonatal pink eye caused by sexually transmitted infections, like gonorrhea or chlamydia, can be very serious. If you are pregnant and think you may have a sexually transmitted infection, visit your healthcare provider for testing and treatment. If you don't know whether you have a sexually transmitted infection but have recently given birth and your newborn shows signs of pink eye, visit your child's healthcare provider right away.

Most hospitals are required by state law to put drops or ointment in a newborn's eyes to prevent pink eye.

Vernal Keratoconjunctivitis

What Is Vernal Keratoconjunctivitis?

Vernal keratoconjunctivitis (VKC) is a chronic, severe allergy that affects the surfaces of the eyes. It most commonly occurs in boys living in warm, dry climates. Attacks associated with VKC are common in the spring (hence the name "vernal") and summer but often reoccur in the winter. Signs and symptoms usually begin before 10 years of age and may include hard, cobblestone-like bumps (papillae) on the upper eyelid; sensitivity to light; redness; sticky mucus discharge; and involuntary blinking or spasms of the eyelid (blepharospasm). The condition usually subsides at the onset of puberty. It is caused by a hypersensitivity (allergic reaction) to airborne-allergens. Management focuses on preventing "flare ups" and relieving the symptoms of the condition.

> Vernal keratoconjunctivitis (VKC) is a fairly common disease in hot, dry environments, representing as much as 3 percent of severe ophthalmic diseases and up to 33 percent of all eye pathology seen among young patients in eye clinics in Central Africa.
>
> *(Source: "Pneumonia," ClinicalTrials.gov, National Institutes of Health (NIH).)*

What Is The Incidence Of Vernal Keratoconjunctivitis?

A review of available literature currently does not yield information about the overall incidence (the rate of occurrence of new cases) of vernal keratoconjunctivitis (VKC). VKC has a wide geographical distribution and varying prevalence (the total number of cases in a given population at a specific time) has been reported in different ethnic groups. It is most common in young males living in dry, hot climates such as in Mediterranean areas, central and west Africa, the Middle East, Japan, the Indian subcontinent and South America. It is also seen in Western Europe (including the UK and Sweden), Australia and North America—although the prevalence in these countries has probably increased due to migration of more susceptible populations.

One survey suggests VKC may have a prevalence rate of 3.2 per 10,000 individuals in Western Europe. Another study involving over 400 affected individuals only in an area of Northern Italy reported that the average incidence independent of gender and age was 1 in

100,000 new cases. The authors reported a higher rate in males under 16 years of age (10 in 100,000) compared with females (4.2 in 100,000).

How Might Vernal Keratoconjunctivitis Be Treated?

Management of vernal keratoconjunctivitis (VKC) focuses on preventing allergic attacks as well as relieving the signs and symptoms of the condition. It is often recommended that affected individuals try to avoid the agent that causes the allergy (if possible); wear dark sunglasses in the daytime; avoid dust; and stay inside on hot afternoons. Eye drops that affect the amount of histamine released by immune system cells (called mast cell stabilizers) may be used at the beginning of the season or at the first sign of a "flare-up" to prevent severe symptoms; however, they are not considered effective at relieving symptoms. Topical eye drops are generally preferred as the first source of treatment. Cold compresses, artificial tears, ointments and/or topical antihistamines may help. Nonsteroid anti-inflammatory drugs (NSAIDs) may relieve symptoms in moderate cases; topical steroids are typically only used for more severe cases because long-term use can cause glaucoma.

A few prescription drugs may also be available for the treatment of VKC; these include cromolyn sodium, lodoxamide tromethamine and Levocabastine. Oral administration of montelukast, a drug usually prescribed for asthma, has also been shown to be an effective treatment of VKC.

What Is The Prognosis For Individuals With Vernal Keratoconjunctivitis?

Vernal keratoconjunctivitis (VKC) generally resolves spontaneously after puberty without any further symptoms or visual complications. However, the development of corneal ulcers (in approximately 9.7 percent of affected individuals), cataract or glaucoma can potentially cause permanent vision loss. Beginning treatment immediately after receiving the diagnosis of VKC is very important because the longer an individual has complications from the disease, the greater the chances of developing cataracts or permanent blindness. It has been reported that the size of the papillae is directly related to the probability of persistence or worsening of symptoms (i.e., the larger the papillae, the worse the prognosis is). It has also been reported that the bulbar forms of VKC have a worse long-term prognosis than the tarsal forms.

Chapter 18

Contact Dermatitis And Latex Allergy

What Is Contact Dermatitis?

Occupationally related contact dermatitis can develop from frequent and repeated use of hand hygiene products, exposure to chemicals, and glove use. Contact dermatitis is classified as either irritant or allergic. Irritant contact dermatitis is common, nonallergic, and develops as dry, itchy, irritated areas on the skin around the area of contact. By comparison, allergic contact dermatitis (type IV hypersensitivity) can result from exposure to accelerators and other chemicals used in the manufacture of rubber gloves as well as from exposure to other chemicals found in the dental practice setting. Allergic contact dermatitis often manifests as a rash beginning hours after contact and, like irritant dermatitis, is usually confined to the areas of contact.

Call Your Doctor If...

- Your rash is so uncomfortable or painful it interferes with daily activities or sleep.
- The rash is on your face.
- Your rash looks worrisome or seems infected.

About This Chapter: Text beginning with the heading "What Is Contact Dermatitis?" is excerpted from "Frequently Asked Questions—Contact Dermatitis And Latex Allergy," Centers for Disease Control and Prevention (CDC), July 10, 2013. Reviewed November 2017; Text under the heading "Treatment" is excerpted from "Red, Itchy Rash?" *NIH News in Health*, National Institutes of Health (NIH), April 2012. Reviewed November 2017.

- You break out in a rash after taking a new medication.
- Your rash lasts for several days.

Your skin is your protection. It's not just the covering that keeps your body in; it's also your first line of defense against germs and chemicals. Take care of your skin so your skin can take care of you.

(Source: "Red, Itchy Rash? Get The Skinny On Dermatitis," NIH News in Health, *National Institutes of Health (NIH).)*

What Is Latex Allergy?

Latex allergy (type I hypersensitivity to latex proteins) can be a more serious systemic allergic reaction. It usually begins within minutes of exposure but can sometimes occur hours later. It produces varied symptoms, which commonly include runny nose, sneezing, itchy eyes, scratchy throat, hives, and itchy burning sensations. However, it can involve more severe symptoms including asthma marked by difficult breathing, coughing spells, and wheezing; cardiovascular and gastrointestinal ailments; and in rare cases, anaphylaxis and death.

What Are The Categories Of Glove-Associated Skin Reactions?

Table 18.1. Categories Of Glove-Associated Skin Reactions

	Irritant Contact Dermatitis	**Allergic Contact Dermatitis (Type IV [Delayed] Hypersensitivity)**	**Latex Allergy (Type I [Immediate] Hypersensitivity Or Natural Rubber Latex (NRL) Protein Allergy)**
Causative Agents	Toxic chemicals (e.g., biocides, detergents); excessive perspiration; irritating chemicals used in hand products and in glove manufacture	Accelerators and other chemicals used in glove manufacture; sterilants and disinfectants (e.g., glutaraldehyde); bonding agents (e.g., methracrylates); local anesthetics	Latex proteins from *Hevea brasiliensis* (rubber tree)

Table 18.1. Continued

	Irritant Contact Dermatitis	Allergic Contact Dermatitis (Type IV [Delayed] Hypersensitivity)	Latex Allergy (Type I [Immediate] Hypersensitivity Or Natural Rubber Latex (NRL) Protein Allergy)
Reactions	Skin reactions usually confined to the area of contact	Skin reactions usually confined to the area of contact	Skin and systemic reactions can occur as soon as 2–3 minutes, or as long as several hours after skin or mucous membrane contact with the protein allergens
	Acute: Red, dry, itchy irritated areas	**Acute:** Itchy, red rash, small blisters	**Acute:** Hives, swelling, runny nose, nausea, abdominal cramps, dizziness, low blood pressure, bronchospasm, anaphylaxis (shock)
	Chronic: Dry, thickened skin, crusting, deep painful cracking, scabbing sores, peeling	**Chronic:** Dry thickened skin, crusting, scabbing sores, vesicles, peeling (appears 4–96 hours after exposure)	**Chronic:** As above, increased potential for extensive, more severe reaction
Diagnosis	By medical history, symptoms, and exclusion of Type IV and Type I hypersensitivity. Not an allergic reaction	By medical history, symptoms, and skin patch test	By medical history, symptoms, and skin-prick or blood test

Dental healthcare personnel experiencing contact dermatitis or latex allergy symptoms should seek a definitive diagnosis by an experienced healthcare professional (e.g., dermatologist, allergist) to determine the specific etiology and appropriate treatment for their condition, as well as to determine what work restrictions or accommodations may be necessary.

Why Are Powder-Free Gloves Recommended?

Proteins responsible for latex allergies are attached to glove powder. When powdered gloves are worn, more latex protein reaches the skin. Also, when gloves are put on or removed, particles of latex protein powder become aerosolized and can be inhaled, contacting mucous membranes. As a result, allergic dental healthcare personnel and patients can experience symptoms related to cutaneous, respiratory, and conjunctival exposure. Dental healthcare personnel can become sensitized to latex proteins after repeated exposure. Work areas where only powder-free, low-allergen (i.e., reduced-protein) gloves are used show low or undetectable amounts of allergy-causing proteins.

Treatment

Mild cases of allergic contact dermatitis usually disappear after a few days or weeks. But if the rash persists, is extremely uncomfortable or occurs on the face, it's important to see a physician. A doctor can prescribe medications that will tone down the immune reaction in the skin. This eases swelling and itching and will protect your eyes and face.

The immune cells of the skin can also produce rashes when they react to invading germs—like bacteria, fungi and viruses. Bacterial and viral infections within your body can cause your skin to break out in spots as well. The chickenpox virus, for example, can cause itchy spots in children. Years later, in older adults, the same virus may reappear as shingles, bringing a painful rash and high fever. Vaccines can prevent several rash-causing diseases, including chickenpox, shingles and measles.

Certain drugs, including antibiotics like amoxicillin, may also cause itchy skin rashes. If you're allergic to a drug, a rash can be the first sign of a serious reaction. As with other allergies, a reaction to a drug may not occur the first time you take it. It could show up after several uses. Not all drug rashes are due to an allergy, however. If you break out in itchy spots after starting a new drug prescription, contact your doctor right away.

While most rashes get better with time, some can last a lifetime. Psoriasis, a condition where skin cells buildup into thick red patches, tends to run in families. "It's a complex genetic disease, in that there's not one gene that causes psoriasis but many," says Katz. Even though none of these genes alone has a great effect on the disease, knowing which genes are involved can help researchers design potential new treatments. Other long-term diseases that can produce rashes include autoimmune diseases, such as lupus, and some forms of cancer.

If you notice an itchy or painful rash on your skin, think twice before going to the drugstore and getting some cream if you don't know the cause. "The creams that you buy can produce problems that make your original problem even worse," Katz says. Because rashes can be caused by many different things—bacteria, viruses, drugs, allergies, genetic disorders, and even light—it's important to figure out what kind of dermatitis you have.

"If you have any significant rash, you should see a dermatologist," says Katz. A dermatologist, or skin doctor, is specially trained to figure out what's causing a rash and help you get the right treatment.

Chapter 19

Atopic Dermatitis (Eczema)

Atopic dermatitis is a skin disease. When a person has this disease the skin becomes extremely itchy. Scratching leads to redness, swelling, cracking, "weeping" clear fluid, crusting, and scaling. Often, the skin gets worse (flares), and then it improves or clears up (remissions).

Atopic dermatitis is the most common kind of eczema, a term that describes many kinds of skin problems.

- Atopic dermatitis is the most common kind of eczema, a term that describes many kinds of skin problems.

- The disease causes the skin to become very itchy. Scratching leads to redness, swelling, cracking, "weeping" clear fluid, crusting, and scaling.

- Often, the skin gets worse (flares), and then it improves or clears up (remissions).

- Treatment usually includes medications, proper skin care, and avoiding things that cause allergies.

- Avoid scratching itchy skin, which only worsens symptoms.

- You should not get the smallpox vaccine if you have atopic dermatitis.

About This Chapter: This chapter includes text excerpted from "Atopic Dermatitis," National Institute of Arthritis and Musculoskeletal and Skin Diseases (NIAMS), July 31, 2016.

Who Gets It?

Atopic dermatitis is most common in babies and children. But it can happen to anyone. People who live in cities and dry climates may be more likely to get this disease.

You can't "catch" the disease or give it to other people.

What Are The Symptoms?

The most common symptoms of atopic dermatitis are:

- Dry and itchy skin.

- Rashes on the face, inside the elbows, behind the knees, and on the hands and feet.

Scratching the skin can cause:

- Redness

- Swelling

- Cracking

- "Weeping" clear fluid

- Crusting

- Thick skin

- Scaling

Complications

A major health risk associated with atopic dermatitis is skin colonization or infection by bacteria such as *Staphylococcus aureus*. Sixty to 90 percent of people with atopic dermatitis are likely to have staph bacteria on their skin. Many eventually develop infection, which worsens the atopic dermatitis.

People with atopic dermatitis are highly vulnerable to certain viral infections of the skin. For example, if infected with herpes simplex virus, they can develop a severe skin condition called atopic dermatitis with eczema herpeticum.

(Source: "Eczema (Atopic Dermatitis) Complications," National Institute of Allergy and Infectious Diseases (NIAID).)

What Causes It?

No one knows what causes atopic dermatitis. It is probably passed down from your parents (genetics). Your environment can also trigger symptoms. Stress can make the condition worse, but it does not cause the disease.

Is There A Test?

Currently, there is no single test to diagnose atopic dermatitis, but your doctor may:

- Ask you about your medical history, including:

    - Your family history of allergies.

    - Whether you also have diseases such as hay fever or asthma.

    - Exposure to irritants, such as:

        - Wool or synthetic fibers.

        - Soaps and detergents.

        - Some perfumes and cosmetics.

        - Substances such as chlorine, mineral oil, or solvents.

        - Dust or sand.

        - Cigarette smoke.

    - Sleep problems.

    - Foods that seem to be related to skin flares.

    - Previous treatments for skin-related symptoms.

    - Use of steroids or other medications.

- Identify factors that may trigger flares of atopic dermatitis by pricking the skin with a needle that contains something that you might be allergic to (in small amounts).

Your doctor may need to see you several times to diagnose you. In some cases, your family doctor or pediatrician may refer you to a dermatologist (doctor specializing in skin disorders) or allergist (allergy specialist) for further evaluation.

How Is It Treated?

The goals in treating atopic dermatitis are to heal the skin and prevent flares. You should watch for changes in the skin to find out what treatments help the most.

Treatments can include:

- Medications:

    - Skin creams or ointments that control swelling and lower allergic reactions.

    - Corticosteroids.

    - Antibiotics to treat infections caused by bacteria.

    - Antihistamines that make people sleepy to help stop nighttime scratching.

    - Drugs that suppress the immune system.

- Light therapy.

- Skin care that helps heal the skin and keep it healthy.

- Avoiding things that cause an allergic reaction.

Who Treats It?

Atopic dermatitis may be treated by:

- Family doctors or pediatricians, who can help diagnosis the disease or refer you to specialists.
- Dermatologists, who specialize in skin disorders.
- Allergists, who specialize in allergies.

Living With It

Besides medications, there are a number of things you can do to help control your atopic dermatitis.

- Skin care: Sticking with a daily skin care routine can prevent flares. Skin care should include:

    - Lukewarm baths to cleanse and moisturize the skin without drying it out.

    - Using mild bar soap or nonsoap cleanser.

- Air-drying the skin after bathing, or gently patting it dry.

- A moisturizer to seal in the water after bathing. Use creams and ointments and avoid lotions with high water or alcohol content.

- Protecting the skin from rough clothing, such as wool or man-made fibers.

- Stay away from things you are allergic to, such as:
  - Dust mites:
    - Put mattresses and pillows inside special dust-proof covers.
    - Wash sheets, blankets, and bed covers often using hot water.
    - Remove carpets.
  - Molds.
  - Pollen.
  - Cat or dog dander.
  - Some perfumes and makeups.
  - Certain foods such as eggs, peanuts, milk, fish, soy products, or wheat. You should change your diet to avoid any foods you are allergic to.

- Stress management and relaxation techniques to decrease numbers of flares. Talking to family, friends, health professionals, and support groups can help.

- Prevent scratching or rubbing, which irritates the skin, increases swelling, and actually increases itchiness. Keep your child's fingernails short to help reduce scratching.

Atopic dermatitis and vaccination against smallpox. People with atopic dermatitis should not get the smallpox vaccine. It may cause serious problems in people with atopic dermatitis.

Points To Remember About Atopic Dermatitis

- Atopic dermatitis is the most common kind of eczema, a term that describes many kinds of skin problems.

- The disease causes the skin to become very itchy. Scratching leads to redness, swelling, cracking, "weeping" clear fluid, crusting, and scaling.

- Often, the skin gets worse (flares), and then it improves or clears up (remissions).

- Treatment usually includes medications, proper skin care, and avoiding things that cause allergies.

- Avoid scratching itchy skin, which only worsens symptoms.

- You should not get the smallpox vaccine if you have atopic dermatitis.

Chapter 20

Urticaria (Hives)

What Is Urticaria?

Urticaria, commonly known as hives, is a condition in which itchy, swollen red wheals, or welts of different sizes appear on the skin. Although there are many possible causes of hives, they most commonly result from an allergic reaction to food or drugs. Hives can last from several minutes to several hours, or in some cases several weeks. They can be itchy, painful, and sometimes cause a burning sensation. Hives may form in one small area on the surface of the skin, or on a larger area of the body. They affect one out of every five people at some point in life.

There are two distinct types of urticaria, acute and chronic. Acute urticaria typically lasts for less than six weeks. The rashes appear suddenly and disappear within a short period of time. Chronic hives, on the other hand, last for more than six weeks and sometimes for months. Although the condition is not dangerous, it can cause considerable discomfort. Angioedema is another form of hives in which the swelling occurs beneath the surface of the skin, often around the eyes and lips.

> Hives are generally not life threatening and do not have long-term health effects. However, when breathing difficulties, dizziness, and swelling of the throat or tongue occur along with an eruption of hives on the skin, it could signal anaphylaxis—a severe, life-threatening allergic reaction—and emergency medical care must be sought.

About This Chapter: "Urticaria (Hives)," © 2016 Omnigraphics. Reviewed November 2017.

Causes And Treatment

Hives usually occur as a symptom of allergic reactions, when the body's immune system releases histamines and other chemicals into the bloodstream. Hives may be triggered by contact with a variety of common allergens, including foods, drugs, latex, pollen, insect bites, or dust mites. Urticaria may also occur as a result of bacterial and viral infections; immunizations; disease conditions such as vasculitis and lupus; adverse reactions to blood transfusions; or skin contact with plants such as poison ivy. In some cases, hives may also be caused by external triggers such as exercise, emotional stress, heat and cold, and sun exposure.

While the cause of hives may be obvious in people with known allergies, other people may need to undergo medical testing by specialists to identify the cause. In some people with chronic hives, the underlying cause may be difficult to find. It may be helpful to keep a diary of symptoms, noting the conditions under which they occur and improve. This information can help people identify and avoid any factors that can trigger the condition.

As the first course of treatment for hives, a healthcare provider will usually prescribe antihistamine medication to negate the effects of histamines released into the bloodstream. Corticosteroids may be prescribed if the symptoms are severe. If the patient experiences hives as part of a severe allergic reaction and has symptoms of anaphylaxis, they will require an immediate shot of epinephrine. Anti-itch medications or salves may also be prescribed to provide relief from itching. Applying wet compresses or taking a cool bath with baking soda or oatmeal sprinkled in the water can also help relieve symptoms of hives.

Vibratory urticaria is a condition in which exposing the skin to vibration, repetitive stretching, or friction results in allergy symptoms such as hives (urticaria), swelling (angioedema), redness (erythema), and itching (pruritus) in the affected area. The reaction can be brought on by towel drying, hand clapping, running, a bumpy ride in a vehicle, or other repetitive stimulation. Headaches, fatigue, faintness, blurry vision, a metallic taste in the mouth, facial flushing, and more widespread swelling (especially of the face) can also occur during these episodes, especially if the stimulation is extreme or prolonged. The reaction occurs within a few minutes of the stimulation and generally lasts up to an hour. Affected individuals can have several episodes per day.

(Source: "Vibratory Urticaria," Genetics Home Reference (GHR), National Institutes of Health (NIH)

References

1. Cole, Gary W. "Hives (Urticaria and Angiodema)," MedicineNet, n.d.

2. "Hives (Urticaria)," American College of Allergy, Asthma, and Immunology, 2014.

3. "Hives," MedlinePlus, U.S. National Library of Medicine, September 8, 2014.

Chapter 21

Anaphylaxis And Exercise-Induced Anaphylaxis

Anaphylaxis

Anaphylaxis is a serious allergic reaction. It can begin very quickly, and symptoms may be life-threatening. The most common causes are reactions to foods (especially peanuts), medications, and stinging insects. Other causes include exercise and exposure to latex. Sometimes no cause can be found.

> Anaphylaxis occurs when mast cells release large quantities of chemicals (histamines, prostaglandins, and leukotrienes) that cause blood vessels to leak, bronchial tissues to swell and blood pressure to drop. Resulting conditions such as shock and unconsciousness usually resolve in most people treated with epinephrine (adrenaline) and first aid measures. In rare cases, however, death may occur.
>
> *(Source: "Abnormal Immune Cells May Cause Unprovoked Anaphylaxis," National Institutes of Health (NIH).)*

It can affect many organs:

- **Skin:** itching, hives, redness, swelling

- **Nose:** sneezing, stuffy nose, runny nose

About This Chapter: Text under the heading "Anaphylaxis" is excerpted from "Anaphylaxis," National Institute of Allergy and Infectious Diseases (NIAID), September 21, 2016; Text under the heading "Exercise-Induced Anaphylaxis" is excerpted from "Exercise-Induced Anaphylaxis," Genetic and Rare Diseases Information Center (GARD), National Center for Advancing Translational Sciences (NCATS), October 12, 2016.

- **Mouth:** itching, swelling of the lips or tongue
- **Throat:** itching, tightness, trouble swallowing, swelling of the back of the throat
- **Chest:** shortness of breath, coughing, wheezing, chest pain or tightness
- **Heart:** weak pulse, passing out, shock
- **Gastrointestinal tract:** vomiting, diarrhea, cramps
- **Nervous system:** dizziness or fainting

If someone is having a serious allergic reaction, call 9-1-1. If an auto-injector is available, give the person the injection right away.

Exercise-Induced Anaphylaxis

Exercise-induced anaphylaxis (EIAn) is a rare disorder in which anaphylaxis occurs in association with physical activity. Food-dependent exercise-induced anaphylaxis is a subset of this disorder in which symptoms develop if exertion takes place within a few hours of eating a specific food. In the case of food-dependent exercise-induced anaphylaxis, neither the food nor the exercise alone is enough to cause anaphylaxis.

Vigorous forms of physical activity, such as jogging, are more commonly associated with exercise-induced anaphylaxis, although lower levels of exertion (e.g., walking and yard work) are also capable of triggering attacks. However, the condition can be unpredictable; a given level of exercise may cause an episode on one occasion but not another.

Symptoms of exercise-induced anaphylaxis may include itching, hives (urticaria), flushing, extreme fatigue, and wheezing. Affected individuals may also experience nausea, abdominal cramping, and diarrhea. Continuing the physical activity causes the symptoms to become worse. However, if the individual stops the activity when the symptoms first appear, there is usually improvement within minutes. In most cases, these conditions are sporadic, though familial cases have been reported.

Treatment

Prevention remains the best treatment for patients with exercise-induced anaphylaxis. Management should include education about safe conditions for exercise, identification and avoidance of offending foods, the importance of stopping exercise immediately if symptoms develop, the appropriate use of epinephrine, and the importance of having epinephrine available at all times.

Patients may also be advised to wear a medical alert bracelet with instructions on the use of epinephrine. The following factors may increase the risk of an exercise-induced attack and are often considered cofactors:

- nonsteroidal anti-inflammatory drugs (NSAIDs),

- alcohol,

- certain phases of the menstrual cycle,

- temperature extremes, and

- seasonal pollen exposure.

As a result, patients may be advised to minimize their exposure to these risk factors.

Prognosis

The prognosis for patients with exercise-induced anaphylaxis is generally favorable. Most patients experience fewer and less severe attacks over time. Although rare, fatalities have been reported, though many of these cases had extenuating circumstances. No cure for this disorder exists. With appropriate lifestyle changes, however, patients may be able to reduce or eliminate episodes of anaphylaxis, and prompt intervention can shorten those episodes that do occur.

Chapter 22

Climate Change And Respiratory Allergies

Climate change is expected to affect air quality through several pathways, including production and allergenicity of allergens and increase regional concentrations of ozone, fine particles, and dust. Some of these pollutants can directly cause respiratory disease or exacerbate existing conditions in susceptible populations, such as children or the elderly. Some of the impacts that climate change can have on air quality include:

Health Impacts

- Increase ground level ozone and fine particle concentrations, which can trigger a variety of reactions including chest pains, coughing, throat irritation, and congestion, as well as reduce lung function and cause inflammation of the lungs.

- Increase carbon dioxide concentrations and temperatures, thereby affecting the timing of aeroallergen distribution and amplifying the allergenicity of pollen and mold spores.

- Increase precipitation in some areas leading to an increase in mold spores.

- Increase in rate of ozone formation due to higher temperatures and increased sunlight.

- Increase the frequency of droughts, leading to increased dust and particulate matter.

About This Chapter: This chapter includes text excerpted from "Asthma, Respiratory Allergies And Airway Diseases," National Institute of Environmental Health Sciences (NIEHS), August 24, 2017.

Adaptation And Mitigation

- Mitigating short-lived contamination species that both air pollutants and greenhouse gases, such as ozone or black carbon. Examples include urban tree covers or rooftop gardens in urban settings.

- Decreasing the use of vehicle miles traveled to reduce ozone precursors.

- Utilizing alternative transportation options, such as walking or biking, which have the co-benefit of reducing emissions while increasing cardiovascular fitness and contributing to weight loss. However, these activities also have the potential to increase exposure to harmful outdoor air pollutants, particularly in urban areas.

- Increasing the use of air conditioning can alleviate the health effects of exposure to chronic or acute heat. However, this can potentially result in higher greenhouse gas emissions depending on the method of power generation.

Part Three
Food Allergies And Intolerances

Chapter 23

Food Allergies: What You Need To Know

A food allergy is a potentially serious response to consuming certain foods or food additives. For those who are sensitive, a reaction can occur within minutes or hours, and symptoms can range from mild to life threatening.

(Source: "Allergies And Food Safety," U.S. Department of Agriculture (USDA).)

Each year, millions of Americans have allergic reactions to food. Although most food allergies cause relatively mild and minor symptoms, some food allergies can cause severe reactions, and may even be life-threatening.

There is no cure for food allergies. Strict avoidance of food allergens—and early recognition and management of allergic reactions to food—are important measures to prevent serious health consequences.

What Are Major Food Allergens?

While more than 160 foods can cause allergic reactions in people with food allergies, the law identifies the eight most common allergenic foods. These foods account for 90 percent of food allergic reactions, and are the food sources from which many other ingredients are derived.

About This Chapter: This chapter includes text excerpted from "Food—Food Allergies: What You Need To Know," U.S. Food and Drug Administration (FDA), April 5, 2017.

The eight foods identified by the law are:

1. Milk

2. Eggs

3. Fish (e.g., bass, flounder, cod)

4. Crustacean shellfish (e.g., crab, lobster, shrimp)

5. Tree nuts (e.g., almonds, walnuts, pecans)

6. Peanuts

7. Wheat

8. Soybeans

These eight foods, and any ingredient that contains protein derived from one or more of them, are designated as "major food allergens" by Food Allergen Labeling and Consumer Protection Act (FALCPA).

How Major Food Allergens Are Listed

The law requires that food labels identify the food source names of all major food allergens used to make the food. This requirement is met if the common or usual name of an ingredient (e.g., buttermilk) that is a major food allergen already identifies that allergen food source name (i.e., milk). Otherwise, the allergen food source name must be declared at least once on the food label in one of two ways.

The name of the food source of a major food allergen must appear:

1. **In parentheses** following the name of the ingredient.

    Examples: "lecithin (soy)," "flour (wheat)," and "whey (milk)"

    — OR —

2. **Immediately after or next to** the list of ingredients in a "contains" statement.

    Example: "Contains Wheat, Milk, and Soy."

Severe Food Allergies Can Be Life-Threatening

Following ingestion of a food allergen(s), a person with food allergies can experience a severe, life-threatening allergic reaction called anaphylaxis.

This can lead to:

- constricted airways in the lungs

- severe lowering of blood pressure and shock ("anaphylactic shock")

- suffocation by swelling of the throat

Each year in the United States, it is estimated that anaphylaxis to food results in:
- 30,000 emergency room visits
- 2,000 hospitalizations
- 150 deaths

Prompt administration of epinephrine by auto injector (e.g., Epi-pen) during early symptoms of anaphylaxis may help prevent these serious consequences.

Know The Symptoms

Symptoms of food allergies typically appear from within a few minutes to 2 hours after a person has eaten the food to which he or she is allergic.

Allergic reactions can include:

- Hives

- Flushed skin or rash

- Tingling or itchy sensation in the mouth

- Face, tongue, or lip swelling

- Vomiting and/or diarrhea

- Abdominal cramps

- Coughing or wheezing

- Dizziness and/or lightheadedness

- Swelling of the throat and vocal cords

- Difficulty breathing

- Loss of consciousness

> ## Mild Symptoms Can Become More Severe
> Initially mild symptoms that occur after ingesting a food allergen are not always a measure of mild severity. In fact, if not treated promptly, these symptoms can become more serious in a very short amount of time, and could lead to anaphylaxis.

About Other Allergens

Persons may still be allergic to—and have serious reactions to—foods other than the eight foods identified by the law. So, always be sure to read the food label's ingredient list carefully to avoid the food allergens in question.

What To Do If Symptoms Occur

The appearance of symptoms after eating food may be a sign of a food allergy. The food(s) that caused these symptoms should be avoided, and the affected person, should contact a doctor or healthcare provider for appropriate testing and evaluation.

- Persons found to have a food allergy should be taught to read labels and avoid the offending foods. They should also be taught, in case of accidental ingestion, to recognize the early symptoms of an allergic reaction, and be properly educated on—and armed with—appropriate treatment measures.

- Persons with a known food allergy who begin experiencing symptoms while, or after, eating a food should initiate treatment immediately, and go to a nearby emergency room if symptoms progress.

FDA's Role: Labeling

To help Americans avoid the health risks posed by food allergens, the U.S. Food and Drug Administration (FDA) enforces the Food Allergen Labeling and Consumer Protection Act of 2004 (the Act). The Act applies to the labeling of foods regulated by FDA, which includes all foods except poultry, most meats, certain egg products, and most alcoholic beverages that are regulated by other Federal agencies. The Act requires that food labels must clearly identify the food source names of any ingredients that are one of the major food allergens or contain any protein derived from a major food allergen.

As a result, food labels help allergic consumers identify offending foods or ingredients so they can more easily avoid them.

Food Allergen "Advisory" Labeling

The Food Allergen Labeling and Consumer Protection Act's (FALCPA) labeling requirements do not apply to the potential or unintentional presence of major food allergens in foods resulting from "cross-contact" situations during manufacturing, e.g., because of shared equipment or processing lines. In the context of food allergens, "cross-contact" occurs when a residue or trace amount of an allergenic food becomes incorporated into another food not intended to contain it. FDA guidance for the food industry states that food allergen advisory statements, e.g., "may contain [allergen]" or "produced in a facility that also uses [allergen]" should not be used as a substitute for adhering to current good manufacturing practices and must be truthful and not misleading. FDA is considering ways to best manage the use of these types of statements by manufacturers to better inform consumers.

Reporting Adverse Effects And Labeling Concerns

If you think that you or a family member has an injury or illness that you believe is associated with having eaten a particular food, including individuals with food allergies and those with celiac disease, contact your healthcare provider immediately.

Individuals can report a problem with a food or its labeling, such as potential misuse of "gluten-free" claims, to FDA in either of these ways:

1. Contact MedWatch, FDA's Safety Information and Adverse Event Reporting Program, at 800-332-1088, or file a MedWatch voluntary report at www.fda.gov/Safety/MedWatch/default.htm.

2. Contact the consumer complaint coordinator in their area. The list of FDA consumer complaint coordinators is available at www.fda.gov/safety/reportaproblem/consumer-complaintcoordinators/default.htm.

Chapter 24

Food Allergy And Related Disorders

In addition to studying common food allergies, such as peanut, milk, and egg allergies, National Institute of Allergy and Infectious Diseases (NIAID) funds research on disorders that are related to, or occur alongside, food allergy. Research related to these increasingly diagnosed conditions may offer insight on treatment and prevention.

Oral Allergy Syndrome

Oral allergy syndrome is an allergic reaction to certain raw fruits and vegetables, such as apples, cherries, kiwis, celery, tomatoes, melons, and bananas. Oral allergy syndrome occurs in people with hay fever, or cold like symptoms caused by allergies. The syndrome is most likely to occur in those allergic to birch, grass, and ragweed pollens because some of the protein allergens in these types of pollen are similar in structure to the proteins of certain fruits.

Those with oral allergy syndrome generally do not experience life-threatening reactions, but they can experience a rash, itching, swelling, and sneezing if they eat or even just hold these raw fruits and vegetables. Similar to the experimental baked food approach to treating other food allergies, symptoms typically do not occur after consuming cooked or baked fruits and vegetables, as cooking or processing fruits and vegetables easily breaks down the proteins that cause oral allergy syndrome.

About This Chapter: Text in this chapter begins with excerpts from "Food Allergy—Characterizing Food Allergy And Addressing Related Disorders," National Institute of Allergy and Infectious Diseases (NIAID), April 26, 2016; Text under the heading "Food Allergy Versus Food Intolerance" is excerpted from "Is It Food Allergy Or Food Intolerance?" U.S. Department of Veterans Affairs (VA), April 17, 2015.

Eosinophilic Esophagitis

Eosinophilic esophagitis, or EoE, is a chronic disease that can be associated with food allergies. It is increasingly being diagnosed in children and adults. EoE is characterized by immune cells called eosinophils building up in the esophagus.

Symptoms of EoE include nausea, vomiting, and abdominal pain after eating. A person may also have symptoms that resemble acid reflux from the stomach, known as heartburn. In older children and adults, EoE can cause more severe symptoms, such as difficulty swallowing solid food, or solid food getting stuck in the esophagus and requiring removal by a physician. In infants, this disease may be associated with failure to thrive.

The National Institute of Allergy and Infectious Diseases (NIAID) funded researchers have found several genes associated with the development of EoE and have evaluated treatment with swallowed anti-inflammatory drugs called corticosteroids. A person diagnosed with EoE is usually tested for food allergies. Oftentimes, those that have both food allergy and EoE can avoid EoE symptoms by avoiding their allergen. NIAID currently funds studies investigating the effectiveness of food avoidance diets and other, experimental approaches to controlling EoE.

Conditions Often Mistaken For Food Allergy

People can feel ill after eating specific foods for reasons other than food allergy. Though these disorders may have some symptoms in common, these illnesses should not be confused with food allergy.

A problem often confused with food allergy is food intolerance, which is also an abnormal response to a food product, but differs from an allergy. A common example is an intolerance to lactose, a sugar found in many milk products that can cause an uncomfortable buildup of gas in the gastrointestinal tract. Gluten intolerance, or celiac disease, occurs when the immune system responds abnormally to gluten, a component of barley, wheat, and rye. However, unlike food allergies, these disorders do not involve Immunoglobulin E (IgE) antibodies. The National Institute of Diabetes and Digestive and Kidney Disorders (NIDDK) currently conducts research on lactose and gluten intolerance.

Foodborne illness, or food poisoning, can also be confused with food allergy because of similar symptoms, such as abdominal cramping. Foodborne illness, however, is caused by microbes, microbial products, and other toxins that can contaminate foods that were improperly preserved or processed.

Food Allergy Versus Food Intolerance

A food allergy occurs when a food you eat abnormally triggers your body's immune system.

Food allergies can range from merely irritating to life threatening.

"Food intolerance" is different from a food allergy. Food intolerance is a reaction to a food that does not involve the body's immune system.

Food Allergy

Sometimes even a very small amount of a food can trigger such a response. The body may respond to the food allergen with such symptoms as digestive problems, hives, or impaired airway.

In some cases, the reaction may be as extreme as to be life threatening, with a reaction called anaphylaxis. Anaphylaxis is a severe whole body reaction to an allergen.

Food Intolerance

While the reaction may feel as if it is a food allergy, if the immune system is not responding, it is food intolerance. Sometimes it is an additive to a food item that may trigger the intolerance symptoms.

Chapter 25

Peanut And Tree Nut Allergies

Peanut allergy is one of the most common food allergies, and its prevalence appears to be increasing. One study indicated that the number of children with peanut allergies tripled between 1997 and 2008 in the United States. Siblings of children who are allergic to peanuts are at a higher risk of developing peanut allergies. Although most peanut allergies last a lifetime, an estimated 20 percent of children outgrow them by the age of six.

Peanuts belong to the legumes family, which also includes soybeans, peas, and lentils. They are different from nuts that grow on trees, such as almonds, walnuts, hazelnuts, cashews, Brazil nuts, and pistachios. However, an estimated 25 to 40 percent of people who are allergic to peanuts are also allergic to tree nuts. As a result, many experts suggest that people who are allergic to peanuts also abstain from eating foods containing tree nuts and seeds.

Peanuts and tree nuts contain structurally similar proteins. In an estimated 1 percent of children and 0.5 percent of adults, exposure to these proteins causes the immune system to overreact and release histamine into the bloodstream, which can trigger a severe, whole-body allergic response called anaphylaxis. The symptoms of anaphylaxis can include:

- Hives

- Swelling and rashes

- Itching

- Swelling of the lips and tongue

About This Chapter: "Peanut And Tree Nut Allergies," © 2016 Omnigraphics. Reviewed November 2017; Text under the heading "Cracking The Peanut Allergy" is excerpted from "Cracking The Peanut Allergy—USDA Program Provides Doctors A Way To Help Children," U.S. Department of Agriculture (USDA), September 27, 2017.

- Constriction of the throat

- Difficulty breathing and swallowing

- Vomiting

- Diarrhea

- Dizziness and fainting

- Drop in blood pressure

Generally, people who are allergic to nuts will develop a reaction within a few minutes of exposure. Anyone who experiences these symptoms should seek medical attention. For mild allergic reactions, the healthcare provider may prescribe antihistamines to subdue the immune response. Severe reactions require immediate treatment with epinephrine (adrenaline), typically administered in an auto-injector. Left untreated, anaphylaxis can be fatal.

Peanuts belong to the legumes family, which also includes soybeans, peas, and lentils. They are different from nuts that grow on trees, such as almonds, walnuts, hazelnuts, cashews, Brazil nuts, and pistachios. However, an estimated 25 to 40 percent of people who are allergic to peanuts are also allergic to tree nuts. As a result, many experts suggest that people who are allergic to peanuts also abstain from eating foods containing tree nuts and seeds.

Peanuts and tree nuts contain structurally similar proteins. In an estimated 1 percent of children and .5 percent of adults, exposure to these proteins causes the immune system to overreact and release histamine into the bloodstream, which can trigger a severe, whole-body allergic response called anaphylaxis. The symptoms of anaphylaxis can include:

- Hives

- Swelling and rashes

- Itching

- Swelling of the lips and tongue

- Constriction of the throat

- Difficulty breathing and swallowing

- Vomiting

- Diarrhea

- Dizziness and fainting

- Drop in blood pressure

Generally, people who are allergic to nuts will develop a reaction within a few minutes of exposure. Anyone who experiences these symptoms should seek medical attention. For mild allergic reactions, the healthcare provider may prescribe antihistamines to subdue the immune response. Severe reactions require immediate treatment with epinephrine (adrenaline), typically administered in an auto-injector. Left untreated, anaphylaxis can be fatal.

Diagnosis And Treatment

Peanut and tree nut allergies can be difficult to diagnose through skin tests or blood tests. When these types of allergies are suspected, the allergist may ask the patient to avoid the food in question for two to four weeks. If the patient's symptoms improve as a result of the food-elimination diet, they are most likely allergic to that specific food. When the results are inconclusive, the allergist may request an oral food challenge. During this test, the patient consumes tiny amounts of peanuts or tree nuts in a controlled environment, with emergency medication and equipment on hand in case they have a severe allergic reaction.

The primary form of treatment for peanut and tree nut allergies is strict avoidance of these foods. Eating foods that contain peanuts or tree nuts is the most common cause of severe allergic reactions. Casual contact with the skin is less likely to trigger a severe reaction, unless the residue is transferred from the skin to the eyes, nose, or mouth. Inhaling peanut fumes does not cause an allergic reaction in most people.

People who are allergic to peanuts and tree nuts should always read food labels carefully to ensure that they do not eat products that contain even trace amounts of nuts. Under U.S. law, food manufacturers are required to note whether their products contain nuts. Many companies also voluntarily note whether products were processed in a facility or with equipment that also handles nuts.

People with peanut and tree nut allergies must also be aware of hidden or unexpected sources of nuts. Some common products that often contain peanuts or tree nuts include baked goods, candy, nougat, pralines, egg rolls, chili sauce, enchilada sauce, and mole sauce. Certain types of food establishments are considered dangerous for individuals with peanut allergies due to the risk of cross-contamination, including bakeries, ice cream shops, and African, Asian, or Mexican restaurants.

References

1. "Peanut Allergy," American College of Allergy, Asthma, and Immunology, 2014.

2. "Peanut Allergy," Food Allergy Research and Education, 2015.

Cracking The Peanut Allergy

Doctors and scientists have discovered a way to reduce the chances of children developing a common and sometimes deadly allergy. Recent studies have found that peanut allergies can be prevented in a high percentage of cases by introducing children to peanut-containing foods while they are still infants.

The revelation was made possible, in part, thanks to the resources provided by the National Peanut Board (NPB), an industry-funded board, established through a research, promotion and information program at the request of peanut producers. The program is overseen by the Promotion and Economics Division of U.S. Department of Agriculture's (USDA) Agricultural Marketing Service, Specialty Crops Program.

With a focus on promoting U.S. grown peanuts, NPB members recognized the increased reporting of peanut allergies among American children, and realized they needed to be part of the solution. The board helped to fund a study called Learning Early About Peanut Allergy (LEAP) that was conducted by researchers at the United Kingdom's Kings College London.

The results of the study were published in the *New England Journal of Medicine*. In the study, up to 86 percent of the infants with a high risk (those with severe eczema, egg allergy, or both) for developing a peanut allergy who ate peanut foods between the ages of 4 and 11 months developed a protective factor that reduced their risk of having the allergy.

To be sure that this protection was long-term and did not simply delay the start of peanut allergies, the researchers conducted a follow-on study. The second study was called LEAP-On. During LEAP-On, the children from the LEAP study who were exposed to peanut foods at an early age were not given peanut foods for 12 months. Researchers found that the protection was indeed long lasting.

In 2008, NPB provided funding to help initiate the early research published in the *Journal of Allergy and Clinical Immunology* that led to the groundbreaking LEAP study and NPB continues to support this work. This research has contributed to the American Academy of Pediatrics (AAP) recommending early introduction of peanut protein for infants who are at increased risk of developing the allergy. In January, the National Institute of Allergy and Infectious Diseases (NIAID) released guidelines for practitioners and caregivers that details when and how to introduce peanut foods safely to prevent peanut allergies. More recently, the FDA acknowledged a qualified health claim linking early peanut introduction and reduced risk of developing peanut allergies.

The collaboration between the board and researchers at the Kings College London (KCL) is a great example of how USDA research and promotion boards can make a difference for people everywhere. In fact, according to the National Institutes of Health (NIH) in a news release about the new guidelines, NIAID Director Anthony S. Fauci, M.D. said, "We expect that widespread implementation of these guidelines by healthcare providers will prevent the development of peanut allergy in many susceptible children and ultimately reduce the prevalence of peanut allergy in the United States."

With this in mind, NPB continues to promote the new guidelines and recommendations for early introduction by educating health professionals, working with influencers, and reaching out to consumers directly.

Parents should always consult with their child's pediatrician to determine the best course of action for treatment of allergies.

Chapter 26

Wheat Allergy

What Is Wheat Allergy?

There are four proteins found in wheat: albumin, globulin, gliadin, and glutenin (also known as gluten). In an individual with a wheat allergy, the immune system develops IgE (immunoglobulin E) antibodies to one or more of these proteins. When the person consumes wheat, the antibodies attack the protein, causing abnormal clinical reactions. These reactions may range from a mild skin rash or runny nose to a severe asthma attack or life-threatening anaphylaxis. Other possible symptoms of wheat allergy include bloated stomach, nausea, vomiting, and diarrhea.

A wheat allergy is different from gluten sensitivity and celiac disease. The majority of wheat allergies involve albumin and globulin. People with gluten sensitivity cannot tolerate gluten, which can be found in grains such as rye and barley in addition to wheat. Celiac disease is a severe form of gluten sensitivity in which the immune system reacts to gluten by producing IgG (immunoglobulin G) antibodies, which cause inflammation in the lining of the small intestine. This inflammation can cause permanent damage to the small intestine and prevent it from absorbing nutrients. For people with celiac disease, the symptoms are generally confined to the abdomen and get worse over time.

Diagnosis And Treatment

Wheat allergy is usually diagnosed by a pinprick skin test or an immunoglobulin blood test. Doctors may also ask the patient to keep a food diary, noting symptoms experienced after eating or eliminating certain foods from their diet. Wheat allergies are most commonly found

About This Chapter: "Wheat Allergy?" © 2016 Omnigraphics. Reviewed November 2017.

in infants and toddlers. In the majority of these cases, the child outgrows the allergy within a few years and wheat can gradually be reintroduced to their diet. A family history of allergies is considered a risk factor for developing a wheat allergy.

Avoidance of wheat-based products is the best treatment for a wheat allergy. Wheat proteins are present in many food items, such as bread, pasta, breakfast cereals, crackers, pretzels, cakes, and some sauces. Wheat proteins are also found in beer, root beer, and gravy. Monosodium glutamate (MSG), used as a flavor enhancer in many foods, is another product in which wheat proteins can be found. The FDA has made it mandatory for food manufacturers to mention "wheat" on the product label if wheat is present in any form. People with wheat allergies must read food labels carefully. It is also important to be aware of cross contamination of food during preparation and clean all surfaces thoroughly.

Wheat products are a staple in many American households. Fortunately, there are a variety of alternative foods that can replace wheat, such as maize, corn, rice, potato, soy, chickpea, tapioca, oats, millets, and quinoa. Wheat-free noodles, crackers, cereals, and other products have become widely available in recent years due to rising demand by people with gluten sensitivity. A dietitian with expertise in food allergies can help people choose among the alternatives.

References

1. Nordqvist, Christian. "What Is Wheat Allergy?" Medical News Today, November 12, 2013.

2. "Wheat Allergy and Sensitivity," Sandwell and West Birmingham Hospitals NHS Trust, July 2014.

Chapter 27

Soy Allergy

What Is Soy Allergy?

Soy is a plant in the pea family. Although it has been a staple in Asian diets for centuries, it has gained popularity in the United States in recent years. Soybeans, the high-protein seeds of the soy plant, contain chemical compounds called isoflavones that have a variety of uses in traditional or folk medicine. Since isoflavones are similar to the female hormone estrogen, soy products have long been used to treat such women's health concerns as menopausal symptoms, osteoporosis, and breast cancer, as well as conditions like high blood pressure, high cholesterol levels, memory loss, and prostate cancer.

Soy is available in the form of dietary supplements. In addition, soybeans can be cooked and eaten or used to make tofu, soymilk, and other foods. Soy is also commonly used as an additive in a wide variety of processed foods, including baked goods, cheese, and pasta.

Symptoms And Diagnosis

Despite its potential health benefits, soy is a fairly common food allergy. Soy allergy occurs when the human immune system overreacts to the protein in soy, causing the body to produce immunoglobulin E (IgE) antibodies. Increased IgE levels trigger the release of histamines and other chemicals that are typically involved in an allergic response. Soy allergy affects approximately 0.4 percent of children in the United States. A majority of children outgrow soy allergy by the age of three or four, however, so it is relatively less common in adults.

About This Chapter: "Soy Allergy," © 2016 Omnigraphics. Reviewed November 2017.

Common Soy Containing Foods

Edamame (green soybeans), miso (soybean pastes), soy nuts, soy milk, soy protein, soy apricot, tamari, and tempeh (fermented soybean products) are some of the soy containing food products. As per U.S. Food and Drug Administration (FDA) regulations under Food Allergen Labeling and Consumer Protection Act (FALCPA), the major eight food allergens that includes soy, should be mentioned in the label of food products in plain language.

Reactions to soy or its derivatives may involve a range of allergic symptoms, from mild skin rashes to wheezing and abdominal cramps. Anaphylaxis—a severe, life-threatening whole-body allergic response—may occur in some people with soy allergy, but it is rather rare. The most common symptoms of a soy allergy are pruritus (itching) around the lips, mouth, face, or other parts of the body; allergic rhinitis (nasal congestion, sneezing, and watery eyes); and nausea, vomiting, and diarrhea.

How The Allergy Is Diagnosed

A soy allergy is initially diagnosed with a skin prick test (SPT), wherein a measured dose of a liquid containing soy protein extract is introduced into the top layer of the skin with a sterile probe. The appearance of a red bump or flare on the skin indicates a sensitivity to soy and helps the allergist make a diagnosis. A blood test may also be done to measure the amount of IgE antibody in the blood.

Avoiding Soy Products

There is no cure for soy allergy. The only way to prevent symptoms from occurring is to exclude soy products from the diet and avoid foods containing soy in any form. Soy is one of the eight common allergens covered under the federal Food Allergen Labeling and Consumer Protection Act (FALCPA). As a result, food manufacturers are required to state on the label whether a product contains soy or has been manufactured in a facility or with equipment that also produces soy-containing products. People with soy allergy should read food labels carefully and avoid ingesting products that contain even traces of soy. If the information on the label is insufficient, they should contact the manufacturer for clarification.

Soy is widely used as an ingredient in commercial foods. In fact, it is estimated that soy plays a role in the production of 20,000 to 30,000 food products, either directly as an ingredient or indirectly as animal feed. Soy fat and oils are used in foods like margarine and mayonnaise.

Soy isolates find use in meat products, soups, sauces, and imitation dairy products. Tofu, which is clotted soymilk, is a popular ingredient in many savory and sweet dishes. Soy meals and soy flour are part of many types of cereals, breads, and pasta. Lecithin, a derivative of soy, is a common additive in a variety of baked food, chocolates, and confections. Most individuals who are allergic to soy can safely tolerate refined soybean oil and lecithin, but they should check with their allergist before consuming these ingredients.

Research On A Hypoallergenic Strain Of Soy

To address growing concerns about food allergies all over the world, scientists have worked to produce a genetically modified (GM) variety of soybean that eliminates P34, the protein in soybeans that is responsible for causing food allergy. They hope to create a "hypoallergenic soy" that will not trigger allergic reactions. Animal studies using the hypoallergenic variety are underway and will serve as a springboard for human trials. Commercial use of this new form of soy is a long way off, however, pending regulatory approvals in countries that are wary of using GM food technology.

References

1. Agricultural Research Service. "Allergic to Certain Foods?" U.S. Department of Agriculture, February 13, 2009.

2. National Food Service Management Institute. "Food Allergy Fact Sheet: Soy Allergies." University of Mississippi, 2012.

Chapter 28

Dark Chocolate And Milk Allergies

If you're allergic to milk and you love dark chocolate, how do you know whether you can indulge in a candy bar without having an allergic reaction? That's what the U.S. Food and Drug Administration (FDA) wanted to learn, especially after receiving reports that consumers had harmful reactions after eating dark chocolate.

Eight foods, and ingredients containing their proteins, are defined as major food allergens. These foods account for 90 percent of all food allergies:

- milk
- egg
- fish, such as bass, flounder, or cod
- crustacean shellfish, such as crab, lobster, or shrimp
- tree nuts, such as almonds, pecans, or walnuts
- wheat
- peanuts
- soybeans

(Source: "Have Food Allergies? Read The Label," U.S. Food and Drug Administration (FDA).)

Milk is a permitted ingredient in dark chocolate, but it is also one of eight major food allergens (substances that can cause reactions that are sometimes dangerous). United States

About This Chapter: This chapter includes text excerpted from "Consumer Updates—What FDA Learned About Dark Chocolate And Milk Allergies," U.S. Food and Drug Administration (FDA), June 19, 2015.

law requires manufacturers to label food products that are major allergens, as well as food products that contain major allergenic ingredients or proteins. Allergens contained in a food product but not named on the label are a leading cause of FDA requests for food recalls, and undeclared milk is the most frequently cited allergen. Chocolates are one of the most common sources of undeclared milk associated with consumer reactions.

FDA tested nearly 100 dark chocolate bars for the presence of milk. In early 2015, the agency issued preliminary findings, and is now releasing more information about its research. The bars tested by FDA were obtained from different parts of the United States, and each bar was unique in terms of product line and/or manufacturer. Bars were divided into categories based on the statements on the labels.

The bottom line? Unfortunately, you can't always tell if dark chocolate contains milk by reading the ingredients list. FDA researchers found that of 94 dark chocolate bars tested, only 6 listed milk as an ingredient. When testing the remaining 88 bars that did not list milk as an ingredient, FDA found that 51 of them actually did contain milk. In fact, the FDA study found milk in 61 percent of all bars tested.

In part, that's because milk can get into a dark chocolate product even when it is not added as an ingredient. Most dark chocolate is produced on equipment that is also used to produce milk chocolate. In these cases, it is possible that traces of milk may inadvertently wind up in the dark chocolate.

Read 'May' As 'Likely'

To inform consumers that dark chocolate products may contain milk even if not intentionally added, many chocolate manufacturers print "advisory" messages on the label. There's quite a variety of advisory messages, such as:

- "may contain milk"

- "may contain dairy"

- "may contain traces of milk"

- "made on equipment shared with milk"

- "processed in a plant that processes dairy"

- "manufactured in a facility that uses milk"

FDA found that milk was present in 3 out of every 4 dark chocolate products with one of these advisory statements. Some products had milk levels as high as those found in products that declared the presence of milk.

150

When the National Confectioners Association (NCA) was asked for its advice, a spokesperson said, "consumers with milk allergies should not consume dark chocolate products that come with advisory statements, since these products may indeed contain milk proteins."

Another problem is that advisory messages may appear to be conflicting if they are accompanied by dairy-free or vegan statements. "Even a consumer who carefully reads the label may be confused by a statement such as "vegan" (which implies that no animal derived products were used) along with an advisory—or "may contain" statement—referring to the presence of milk," says Stefano Luccioli, M.D., a senior medical advisor at FDA.

Not Quite 'Dairy Free'

In addition to these advisory statements, labels for chocolate bars may make other claims. Some say "dairy-free" or "lactose free," but FDA found milk in 15 percent of the dark chocolates with this label. In addition, 25 percent of dark chocolate products labeled only "vegan" were found to contain milk.

No Message Doesn't Mean No Milk

You shouldn't assume that dark chocolate contains no milk if the label does not mention it at all. "Milk allergic consumers should be aware that 33 percent of the dark chocolates with no mention of milk anywhere on the label were, in fact, found to contain milk," says Luccioli.

What Consumers Can Do

1. Consumers who are sensitive or allergic to milk should know that dark chocolate products are a high-risk food if you're highly milk allergic.

2. Start by checking the ingredients list to see if it includes milk.

3. Read all the label statements on dark chocolate products and avoid those with an advisory statement for milk, even if these products feature also other (and conflicting) statements, such as "dairy-free" or "vegan."

4. View even products with dairy-free claims or without any mention of milk with caution, unless the manufacturer is a trusted source and/or uses dedicated equipment for making milk free chocolate products.

"The chocolate industry will continue to make every effort to understand the needs of allergic consumers and communicate the potential presence of milk allergens in dark chocolate through advisory labeling," says Laura Shumow, director of scientific and regulatory affairs at NCA.

FDA is evaluating the study findings and considering options for addressing the issues identified in the study. Further, allergen contamination is included in the preventive and risk-based controls mandated by the FDA Food Safety Modernization Act (FSMA). Under the proposed Preventive Controls for Human Food (PCHF rule) that is scheduled to become final this fall, food manufacturers would be required to implement a food safety plan that identifies safeguards in place to prevent or significantly reduce such hazards as food allergens.

The proposed rule includes provisions to prevent unintended cross contact between foods that contain allergens and those not intended to contain them. Firms covered by the final rule would have from one to three years after the rule becomes final to comply, depending on the size of the firm.

Table 28.1. Milk Detected In Individual Dark Chocolate Products

Label/Package Statement	Total Number Of Dark Chocolate Products	Number And Percent (%) Of Dark Chocolate Products Testing Positive For Milk
Milk (or milk-derived component)	6	6 (100%)
Advisory Statements (alone or combined)	59	44 (75%)
Dairy-free or lactose-free statements alone	13	2 (15%)
Vegan statement alone	4	1 (25%)
No statement regarding milk	12	4 (33%)
TOTAL	94	57 (61%)

1. Some examples of milk components include cream, milk fat, and sodium caseinate.

2. Advisory statements refers to statements regarding the possible presence of milk, such as "may contain milk (or dairy)," "made on equipment shared with milk," "processed in a plant that processes dairy," or "manufactured in a facility that uses milk." This category also includes "may contain traces" statements, as well as advisory statements combined with either a vegan or dairy-free or lactose statement.

3. Lactose-free chocolates are grouped with dairy-free products although the statement "lactose-free" does not necessarily indicate that the product is free from milk. This is because lactose is a "milk sugar," and its removal does not mean that milk proteins are removed as well.

Chapter 29

Seafood Allergy

What Is Seafood Allergy?

A seafood allergy is an abnormal reaction of the human body when it is exposed to proteins found in fish or shellfish. Finned fish and shellfish come from unrelated families of food, so being allergic to fish does not necessarily mean a person will also be allergic to shellfish. The fish family includes an estimated 20,000 species characterized by fins, scales, and bones, such as tuna, salmon, cod, and halibut. The shellfish family is divided into two main types of marine invertebrates: crustaceans (such as shrimp, crab, and lobster); and molluscs (including clams, mussels, oysters, and squid).

Shellfish allergies affect approximately 1 percent of people, making them twice as common as fish allergies, which affect approximately .5 percent of people. Unlike some other types of food allergies, seafood allergies usually develop in adulthood. An estimated 60 percent of people with shellfish allergies and 40 percent of people with fish allergies experience their first reaction as an adult. Seafood allergies tend to be lifelong, and the reactions are likely to be more severe than those associated with most other types of food allergies.

Diagnosing Seafood Allergies

If someone who is allergic to fish or shellfish, the body's immune system mistakenly recognizes proteins from these species as harmful and generates antibodies to fight them as it would fight an infection. When proteins from seafood enter the body—whether through eating fish, touching or handling fish, or breathing in vapors of cooking fish—the body overreacts and

About This Chapter: "Seafood Allergy," © 2016 Omnigraphics. Reviewed November 2017.

releases histamines into the bloodstream. These chemicals produce various symptoms of allergic reactions, such as coughing, throat tightness, wheezing, watery eyes, skin rashes, stomachaches, diarrhea, or vomiting. A more serious manifestation of a seafood allergy is anaphylaxis, in which the person may experience significant difficulty breathing, a drop in blood pressure, lightheadedness, and loss of consciousness. If the person does not receive medical treatment immediately, an anaphylactic reaction can be life threatening.

Anyone who experiences an allergic reaction to seafood should seek medical advice from an allergist/immunologist—a physician specializing in diagnosing and treating allergies. The allergist will conduct a thorough history and physical examination and perform a skin-prick test or a blood test to isolate and identify the type of allergy. Once diagnosed, the patient will receive instructions on how to avoid allergens and what to do if they have an allergic reaction. The allergist may also provide a referral to a dietitian—a medical professional who specializes in dietetics and nutrition—who can offer additional guidance about which foods to avoid and which foods are safe to consume.

Avoiding Seafood

The best treatment for a seafood allergy is to avoid all forms of the allergenic food, whether it is fish or shellfish. For prepared and packaged foods, be sure to read labels thoroughly to avoid buying foods that may contain fish, even if it is not the main ingredient. The U.S. Food and Drug Administration (FDA) has made it mandatory for manufacturers to mention "fish" on the label of foods that contain fish in any form under the Food Allergen Labeling and Consumer Protection Act of 2004. It is important to note that fish proteins may be present in a wide variety of foods, such as Worcestershire sauce, Caesar salad dressing, and some pasta sauces, dips, and even crackers or biscuits.

At home, make sure all surfaces that were used to prepare fish—utensils, cutting boards, countertops, etc.—are thoroughly cleaned before preparing food for an allergic family member. People with a seafood allergy should also stay away from smoke or steam from cooking fish or shellfish as they carry the protein that may cause an allergic reaction.

Avoid going to restaurants that serve seafood. Cross-contamination is a serious possibility in these establishments, so it is best to choose restaurants that do not serve seafood at all. Chinese, Vietnamese, or Thai food preparations have a risk of cross-contamination due to the predominance of fish in these cuisines. Stay away from fish markets and other places where fish is present. Even if an allergist permits a patient to eat certain types of fish or shellfish, it is important to make sure the allowable foods have not been contaminated with allergens from other types of seafood.

Some dietary supplements, like glucosamine—a supplement often prescribed for people with osteoarthritis—may be obtained from the outer coating of crustaceans. As a result, it may provoke a reaction in people allergic to shellfish. Chondroitin sulfate obtained from shark cartilage is another supplement that should be avoided by people with seafood allergies.

For people who experience severe allergic reactions to seafood, a physician may prescribe emergency allergy medication, such as an epinephrine auto-injector, to alleviate symptoms in case of an allergy attack. This medication should be carried at all times and administered at the very first sign of an allergic reaction to avoid life-threatening anaphylaxis.

References

1. "Fish/Seafood Allergy," Allergy UK, March 2012.

2. "Seafood Allergy," Asthma and Allergy Foundation of America, 2005.

Chapter 30

Lactose Intolerance

What Lactose Intolerance?[1]

Does your stomach churn after you drink milk? Do you have diarrhea soon afterward? If so, you may be lactose intolerant.

The National Institute of Diabetes and Digestive and Kidney Diseases (NIDDK) estimates that 30 to 50 million Americans are lactose intolerant.

Being lactose intolerant means you can't digest lactose—the natural sugar found in milk and other dairy products. People who cannot digest lactose have a shortage, or deficiency, of an enzyme called lactase, which is produced in the small intestine. Lactase breaks down milk sugar into two simpler forms of sugar, which are then absorbed into the bloodstream.

> Lactose intolerance is not the same as a milk allergy, says Kavita Dada, Pharm.D., a senior health promotion officer in the U.S. Food and Drug Administration's (FDA's) Division of Drug Information. "For most people with lactase deficiency, it's a discomfort."
>
> People who have trouble digesting lactose can learn which dairy products and other foods they can eat without discomfort and which ones they should avoid.
>
> But a food allergy—an abnormal response to a food triggered by the immune system—can be life threatening. People with food allergies must avoid certain foods altogether. People with food intolerances can often eat small amounts of the offending foods without having symptoms.

This chapter includes text excerpted from documents published by two public domain sources. Text under headings marked 1 are excerpted from "For Consumers—Problems Digesting Dairy Products?" U.S. Food and Drug Administration (FDA), August 30, 2015; Text under headings marked 2 are excerpted from "Calcium," Office of Dietary Supplements (ODS), National Institutes of Health (NIH), November 17, 2016.

Symptoms[1]

When there is not enough lactase to digest the lactose in the foods a person eats or drinks, the person may have:

- gas

- stomach cramps

- bloating

- nausea

- diarrhea

These symptoms typically occur within 30 minutes to two hours after consuming food containing lactose. Some illnesses can cause these same problems, but a healthcare professional can do tests to see if the problems are caused by lactose intolerance or by another condition.

Who Becomes Lactose Intolerant?[1]

Lactose intolerance is more common in some ethnic groups than others. NIDDK estimates that up to 75 percent of all adult African Americans and Native Americans and 90 percent of Asian Americans are lactose intolerant.

As people age, their bodies produce fewer lactase enzymes, so most people don't have symptoms until they are adults.

Most people inherit the condition from their parents. Lactose intolerance is not very common in children under two years of age, unless the child has a lactase deficiency because of an injury to the small intestine. If you think your infant or child may be lactose intolerant, talk to your child's pediatrician.

Managing Lactose Intolerance[1]

There is no treatment to make the body produce more lactase enzyme, but the symptoms of lactose intolerance can be controlled through diet.

Most older children and adults do not have to avoid lactose completely. People have different levels of tolerance to lactose. Some people might be able to have a tablespoon of milk in a cup of coffee with little or no discomfort. Others have reactions that are so bad they stop drinking milk entirely. Some people who cannot drink milk may be able to eat cheese and yogurt—which have less lactose than milk—without symptoms. They may also be able to consume a lactose containing product in smaller amounts at any one time.

Common foods with lactose are:

- milks, including evaporated and condensed
- creams, including light, whipping, and sour
- ice creams
- sherbets
- yogurts
- some cheeses (including cottage cheese)
- butters

Lactose may also be added to some canned, frozen, boxed, and other prepared foods such as:

- breads and other baked goods
- cereals
- mixes for cakes, cookies, pancakes, and biscuits
- instant potatoes, soups, and breakfast drinks
- lunch meats (other than Kosher)
- frozen dinners
- salad dressings
- margarines
- candies and other snacks

Dietary supplements with lactase enzyme are available to help people digest foods that contain lactose. However, FDA has not formally evaluated the effectiveness of these products, and you may want to ask your doctor if these supplements are right for you.

Recommended Dietary Allowances (RDAs) For Calcium[2]

Table 30.1. Recommended Calcium Intake By Age Group

Age	Male	Female	Pregnant	Lactating
0–6 months*	200 mg	200 mg		
7–12 months*	260 mg	260 mg		
1–3 years	700 mg	700 mg		
4–8 years	1,000 mg	1,000 mg		
9–13 years	1,300 mg	1,300 mg		
14–18 years	1,300 mg	1,300 mg	1,300 mg	1,300 mg
19–50 years	1,000 mg	1,000 mg	1,000 mg	1,000 mg
51–70 years	1,000 mg	1,200 mg		
71+ years	1,200 mg	1,200 mg		

Adequate Intake (AI)

Selected Food Sources Of Calcium[2]

Table 30.2. Calcium Content In Common Foods

Food	Milligrams (mg) Per Serving	Percent DV*
Yogurt, plain, low fat, 8 ounces	415	42
Mozzarella, part skim, 1.5 ounces	333	33
Sardines, canned in oil, with bones, 3 ounces	325	33
Yogurt, fruit, low fat, 8 ounces	313–384	31–38
Cheddar cheese, 1.5 ounces	307	31
Milk, nonfat, 8 ounces**	299	30
Soymilk, calcium-fortified, 8 ounces	299	30
Milk, reduced-fat (2% milk fat), 8 ounces	293	29
Milk, buttermilk, lowfat, 8 ounces	284	28
Milk, whole (3.25% milk fat), 8 ounces	276	28
Orange juice, calcium-fortified, 6 ounces	261	26
Tofu, firm, made with calcium sulfate, ½ cup***	253	25
Salmon, pink, canned, solids with bone, 3 ounces	181	18

Table 30.2. Continued

Food	Milligrams (mg) Per Serving	Percent DV*
Cottage cheese, 1% milk fat, 1 cup	138	14
Tofu, soft, made with calcium sulfate, ½ cup***	138	14
Ready-to-eat cereal, calcium-fortified, 1 cup	100–1,000	10–100
Frozen yogurt, vanilla, soft serve, ½ cup	103	10
Turnip greens, fresh, boiled, ½ cup	99	10
Kale, fresh, cooked, 1 cup	94	9
Ice cream, vanilla, ½ cup	84	8
Chinese cabbage, bok choi, raw, shredded, 1 cup	74	7
Bread, white, 1 slice	73	7
Pudding, chocolate, ready to eat, refrigerated, 4 ounces	55	6
Tortilla, corn, ready-to-bake/fry, one 6" diameter	46	5
Tortilla, flour, ready-to-bake/fry, one 6" diameter	32	3
Sour cream, reduced fat, cultured, 2 tablespoons	31	3
Bread, whole-wheat, 1 slice	30	3
Kale, raw, chopped, 1 cup	24	2
Broccoli, raw, ½ cup	21	2
Cheese, cream, regular, 1 tablespoon	14	1

* DV = Daily Value. DVs were developed by the U.S. Food and Drug Administration (FDA) to help consumers compare the nutrient contents among products within the context of a total daily diet. The DV for calcium is 1,000 mg for adults and children aged 4 years and older. Foods providing 20 percent of more of the DV are considered to be high sources of a nutrient, but foods providing lower percentages of the DV also contribute to a healthful diet.

** Calcium content varies slightly by fat content; the more fat, the less calcium the food contains.

*** Calcium content is for tofu processed with a calcium salt. Tofu processed with other salts does not provide significant amounts of calcium.

Look At Labels[1]

"Lactose free" or "lactose reduced" milk and other products are widely available in grocery stores. These products may be fortified to provide the same nutrients as their lactose containing counterparts.

There is no FDA definition for the terms "lactose free" or "lactose reduced," but manufacturers must provide on their food labels information that is truthful and not misleading.

This means a lactose free product should not contain any lactose, and a lactose-reduced product should be one with a meaningful reduction. Therefore, the terms lactose free and lactose reduced have different meanings, and a lactose-reduced product may still contain lactose that could cause symptoms.

Lactose free or lactose-reduced products do not protect a person who is allergic to dairy products from experiencing an allergic reaction. People with milk allergies are allergic to the milk protein, which is still present when the lactose is removed.

Look at the ingredient label. If any of these words are listed, the product probably contains lactose:

- milk
- cream
- butter
- evaporated milk
- condensed milk
- dried milk
- powdered milk
- milk solids
- margarine
- cheese
- whey
- curds

Highly sensitive individuals should also beware of foods labeled "nondairy," such as powdered coffee creamers and whipped toppings. These foods usually contain an ingredient called sodium caseinate, expressed as "caseinate" or "milk derivative" on the label, that may contain low levels of lactose.

Testing For Lactose Intolerance[1]

A doctor can usually determine if you are lactose intolerant by taking a medical history. In some cases, the doctor may perform tests to help confirm the diagnosis. A simple way to test at home is to exclude all lactose containing products from your diet for two weeks to see if the symptoms go away, and then reintroduce them slowly. If the symptoms return, then you most likely are lactose intolerant. But you may still want to see your doctor to make sure that you are lactose intolerant and do not have a milk allergy or another digestive problem.

Tips For Consumers[1]

If you are lactose intolerant, try lactose free milk or dairy products lower in lactose, such as yogurt and cheese. You may be able to consume dairy products in small amounts without symptoms.

Consume milk or other dairy products with other foods. This helps slow down digestion, making it easier for your body to absorb lactose.

If you're eating few or no dairy products, ask your doctor or dietitian if you are getting enough calcium in your diet. You may need to take dietary supplements with calcium to keep your bones healthy.

Are You Getting Enough Calcium?

You may be avoiding dairy products because of lactose intolerance. Or you might have other reasons. But dairy products are a major source of calcium, vitamin D, and other nutrients that are important for your body. If you're avoiding dairy products, you need to take special care to make sure you're getting enough of these nutrients.

Our heart, muscles, and nerves need calcium to work properly. Our bones need it to grow and stay strong. The body also needs vitamin D to absorb calcium. Nutrition surveys have shown that most people in the United States aren't getting the calcium they need. If you're avoiding milk and dairy products, you may be missing out on important sources of calcium and vitamin D.

One of the major reasons people avoid dairy products is lactose intolerance. Lactose is a natural sugar found in milk and other dairy products. You become lactose intolerant if your body doesn't have enough lactase—an enzyme produced in the small intestine that you need to digest lactose. Undigested lactose can cause stomach cramps, gas and diarrhea within 30 minutes to 2 hours after eating something with lactose.

Lactose intolerance isn't common in young children, but many people gradually lose their ability to digest lactose after childhood. That happens more often in some ethnic groups, such as African Americans, Native Americans, Hispanics, and Asians. Most people who don't completely digest lactose have no symptoms and are entirely healthy, but some people do get those uncomfortable symptoms.

Complicating things, some people mistake the symptoms of intestinal disorders, such as Irritable bowel syndrome (IBS) and inflammatory bowel disease (IBD), for lactose intolerance.

> The National Institutes of Health (NIH) convened a "consensus development" conference to review the scientific evidence and develop objective statements about treating lactose intolerance. The panel concluded that there isn't enough scientific evidence to answer many questions about lactose intolerance, including how many people have it, whether it causes serious health effects or how these effects should be treated. More research will be needed to answer these questions.
>
> If you think you or your children are lactose intolerant, studies suggest you may not need to completely eliminate milk or dairy products from your diet. There are several strategies you can try to ensure you get the nutrients you need. These include spreading your dairy intake throughout the day, combining it with other foods, taking nutritional supplements and choosing reduced lactose or nondairy foods rich in the nutrients found in dairy products.
>
> How much calcium and vitamin D you need depends on your age and other factors. If you're avoiding dairy products, talk to your doctor to make sure you meet your nutrient requirements. You can also check out the *Dietary Guidelines for Americans* for recommendations about dietary intake, including dairy or calcium rich foods.
>
> *(Source: "Dairy Dilemma—Are You Getting Enough Calcium?" NIH News in Health, National Institutes of Health (NIH).)*

Raw Milk And Lactose Intolerance[1]

FDA warns consumers not to drink raw, or unpasteurized, milk. "Raw milk advocates claim that pasteurized milk causes lactose intolerance," says John Sheehan, Director of FDA's Division of Plant and Dairy Food Safety. "This is simply not true. All milk, whether raw or pasteurized, contains lactose, and pasteurization does not change the concentration of lactose nor does it convert lactose from one form into another."

Raw milk advocates also claim that raw milk prevents or cures the symptoms of lactose intolerance. Arguing that raw milk contains Bifidobacteria, they claim these microorganisms are beneficial (probiotic) and create their own lactase, which helps people digest the milk.

"This is not true, either," says Sheehan. "Raw milk can contain Bifidobacteria, but when it does, the bacteria come from fecal matter (animal manure) and are not considered probiotic, but instead are regarded as contaminants."

Drinking raw milk will still cause uncomfortable symptoms in people who are correctly diagnosed as being lactose intolerant. But worse than this discomfort are the dangers of raw milk, which can harbor a host of disease causing germs, says Sheehan. "These microorganisms can cause very serious, and sometimes even fatal, disease conditions in humans."

Chapter 31

Egg Allergy

What Is Egg Allergy?

Egg allergy is caused by an inappropriate response of the immune system to the protein component in egg. Egg allergy is one of the most common food allergies, second only to cow's milk allergy, and estimates suggest that it affects around 2 percent of children in the United States. In most cases, the hypersensitivity to the protein present in the albumen (egg white) or the yolk begins in infancy. Although 70 percent of egg allergies disappear by age sixteen, some people may remain allergic to eggs throughout their lives. Egg white allergy is more common than yolk allergy. While some people are allergic to semi-cooked or raw eggs but can tolerate cooked eggs well, there are those who show intolerance to the food whether it is cooked or raw, and whether it includes egg white or yolk.

The mechanism of egg allergy is much the same as in other types of food allergies. An allergic reaction occurs when immunoglobulin E (IgE), a type of antibody used by the body's immune system to fight pathogens, mistakenly recognizes a harmless food component as a harmful invader. The IgE antibodies bind to the egg protein, triggering the release of histamines and other inflammatory chemicals that can set off a series of adverse reactions. The IgE-mediated allergic reaction is rapid and occurs within half an hour of ingesting the food. Non IgE-mediated reactions typically take longer to manifest and their exact mechanism is unclear, although studies have shown that their pathways may involve T-cells, a type of lymphocyte.

Symptoms of egg allergy can vary depending on the degree of sensitivity to the protein. Mild sensitivity may present skin reactions like rashes and hives. In some people, the hypersensitivity may cause respiratory symptoms like wheezing, nasal congestion, or sneezing, as

About This Chapter: "Egg Allergy," © 2016 Omnigraphics. Reviewed November 2017.

well as gastrointestinal symptoms such as vomiting, diarrhea, and abdominal cramping. In a few cases, egg allergy can cause severe, life-threatening anaphylactic reactions, resulting in a drop in blood pressure, increased heart rate, and loss of consciousness. This type of allergic reaction requires immediate administration of the drug epinephrine and emergency care.

Testing For Egg Allergy

The first step in diagnosing an egg allergy involves reviewing the patient's history of symptoms. The allergist may also order a Skin Prick Test (SPT), in which a measured dose of egg protein in a liquid is placed under the skin using a sterile probe. The appearance of a reddish patch or a small swelling (called a "wheal") within the first 20 minutes of administration of the protein indicates an allergic response. The allergist evaluates the degree of sensitivity to egg protein on the basis of the size of the wheal. If the diagnosis is inconclusive, the doctor may ask for a blood test to evaluate the level of allergen-specific serum IgE.

In some cases, however, egg allergy may be difficult to confirm using these initial tests. For instance, the SPT may yield a negative response even though the patient experiences allergy symptoms after ingesting egg. This problem may arise from differences in quality and stability of the allergen extracts used. Likewise, a blood test may indicate the presence of food-specific IgE despite the absence of any allergy symptoms. In such cases, allergists may resort to an oral challenge test that involves a series of trial-and-error procedures. Often recognized as the "gold standard" for food allergy diagnosis, this test involves a period of egg-free diet followed by gradual reintroduction of the suspect food in measured doses. This test has to be done under medical supervision, particularly in patients who have a history of adverse reactions to the food.

Preventing And Treating Egg Allergy

Although many children outgrow it naturally, there is no cure for egg allergy or any other type of food allergy. The only way to prevent allergic reactions to egg products is to completely avoid egg or egg derivatives. This requires a lot of diligence as egg is a versatile ingredient used in a large number of processed foods, including baked foods, desserts, soups, and pasta. People with egg allergy should be vigilant about reading labels and ingredient lists when they shop for food. They must also be careful to check whether there is a possibility that other food may have come in contact with egg during preparation. At restaurants, it may help to tell the waiter about any food sensitivities, as many restaurants today offer allergy-friendly dining.

As with other food allergies, mild to moderate symptoms of egg allergy are usually treated with antihistamines, bronchodilators, or steroids. Severe, anaphylactic reactions are treated with epinephrine, which can reverse symptoms that can be fatal if left untreated. Some vaccines contain egg protein. People with extreme sensitivity to egg protein are advised to take their shots under the supervision of an allergist or in a medical office equipped to deal with any adverse effects.

Eggs are a major source of dietary protein. A registered dietitian can suggest alternatives to egg to ensure that a person on an egg-free diet gets sufficient protein. They can also suggest egg substitutes that can be incorporated into recipes. Some commonly used substitutes in egg-free recipes include: a mix of baking powder, oil, and water; unflavored gelatin; or yeast dissolved in warm water.

References

1. "Egg Allergy," Food Allergy Research and Education, 2015.

2. "Types of Food Allergy: Egg Allergy," American College of Allergy, Asthma, and Immunology, 2013.

Chapter 32

Gluten Intolerance (Celiac Disease)

What Is Celiac Disease?

Celiac disease is a digestive disorder that damages the small intestine. The disease is triggered by eating foods containing gluten. Gluten is a protein found naturally in wheat, barley, and rye, and is common in foods such as bread, pasta, cookies, and cakes. Many prepackaged foods, lip balms and lipsticks, hair and skin products, toothpastes, vitamin and nutrient supplements, and, rarely, medicines, contain gluten.

Celiac disease can be very serious. The disease can cause long-lasting digestive problems and keep your body from getting all the nutrients it needs. Celiac disease can also affect the body outside the intestine.

Celiac disease is different from gluten sensitivity or wheat intolerance. If you have gluten sensitivity, you may have symptoms similar to those of celiac disease, such as abdominal pain and tiredness. Unlike celiac disease, gluten sensitivity does not damage the small intestine.

Celiac disease is also different from a wheat allergy. In both cases, your body's immune system reacts to wheat. However, some symptoms in wheat allergies, such as having itchy eyes or a hard time breathing, are different from celiac disease. Wheat allergies also do not cause long-term damage to the small intestine.

About This Chapter: This chapter includes text excerpted from "Digestive Diseases—Celiac Disease," National Institute of Diabetes and Digestive and Kidney Diseases (NIDDK), June 2016.

Who Is More Likely To Develop Celiac Disease?

Although celiac disease affects children and adults in all parts of the world, the disease is more common in Caucasians and more often diagnosed in females. You are more likely to develop celiac disease if someone in your family has the disease. Celiac disease also is more common among people with certain other diseases, such as Down syndrome, Turner syndrome, and type 1 diabetes.

How Common Is Celiac Disease?
As many as 1 in 141 Americans has celiac disease, although most don't know it.

What Are The Complications Of Celiac Disease?

Long-term complications of celiac disease include:

- malnutrition, a condition in which you don't get enough vitamins, minerals, and other nutrients you need to be healthy

- accelerated osteoporosis or bone softening, known as osteomalacia

- nervous system problems

- problems related to reproduction

Rare complications can include:

- intestinal cancer

- liver diseases

- lymphoma, a cancer of part of the immune system called the lymph system that includes the gut

In rare cases, you may continue to have trouble absorbing nutrients even though you have been following a strict gluten free diet. If you have this condition, called refractory celiac disease, your intestines are severely damaged and can't heal. You may need to receive nutrients through an intravenous (IV).

What Other Health Problems Do People With Celiac Disease Have?

If you have celiac disease, you also may be at risk for:

- Addison disease
- Hashimoto disease
- primary biliary cirrhosis
- type 1 diabetes

What Are The Symptoms Of Celiac Disease?

Most people with celiac disease have one or more symptoms. However, some people with the disease may not have symptoms or feel sick. Sometimes health issues such as surgery, a pregnancy, childbirth, bacterial gastroenteritis, a viral infection, or severe mental stress can trigger celiac disease symptoms.

If you have celiac disease, you may have digestive problems or other symptoms. Digestive symptoms are more common in children and can include:

- bloating, or a feeling of fullness or swelling in the abdomen
- chronic diarrhea
- constipation
- gas
- nausea
- pale, foul-smelling, or fatty stools that float
- stomach pain
- vomiting

For children with celiac disease, being unable to absorb nutrients when they are so important to normal growth and development can lead to:

- damage to the permanent teeth's enamel
- delayed puberty

- failure to thrive in infants

- mood changes or feeling annoyed or impatient

- slowed growth and short height

- weight loss

Celiac disease also can produce a reaction in which your immune system, or your body's natural defense system, attacks healthy cells in your body. This reaction can spread outside your digestive tract to other areas of your body, including your:

- bones

- joints

- nervous system

- skin

- spleen

Depending on how old you are when a doctor diagnoses your celiac disease, some symptoms, such as short height and tooth defects, will not improve.

Dermatitis Herpetiformis

Dermatitis herpetiformis is an itchy, blistering skin rash that usually appears on the elbows, knees, buttocks, back, or scalp. The rash affects about 10 percent of people with celiac disease. The rash can affect people of all ages but is most likely to appear for the first time between the ages of 30 and 40. Men who have the rash also may have oral or, rarely, genital sores. Some people with celiac disease may have the rash and no other symptoms.

Why Are Celiac Disease Symptoms So Varied?

Symptoms of celiac disease vary from person to person. Your symptoms may depend on:

- how long you were breastfed as an infant; some studies have shown that the longer you were breastfed, the later celiac disease symptoms appear

- how much gluten you eat

- how old you were when you started eating gluten

- the amount of damage to your small intestine

- your age—symptoms can vary between young children and adults

People with celiac disease who have no symptoms can still develop complications from the disease over time if they do not get treatment.

What Causes Celiac Disease?

Research suggests that celiac disease only happens to individuals who have particular genes. These genes are common and are carried by about one third of the population. Individuals also have to be eating food that contains gluten to get celiac disease. Researchers do not know exactly what triggers celiac disease in people at risk who eat gluten over a long period of time. Sometimes the disease runs in families. About 10 to 20 percent of close relatives of people with celiac disease also are affected.

Your chances of developing celiac disease increase when you have changes in your genes, or variants. Certain gene variants and other factors, such as things in your environment, can lead to celiac disease.

How Do Doctors Diagnose Celiac Disease?

Celiac disease can be hard to diagnose because some of the symptoms are like symptoms of other diseases, such as irritable bowel syndrome (IBS) and lactose intolerance. Your doctor may diagnose celiac disease with a medical and family history, physical exam, and tests. Tests may include blood tests, genetic tests, and biopsy.

Medical And Family History

Your doctor will ask you for information about your family's health—specifically, if anyone in your family has a history of celiac disease.

Physical Exam

During a physical exam, a doctor most often:

- checks your body for a rash or malnutrition, a condition that arises when you don't get enough vitamins, minerals, and other nutrients you need to be healthy
- listens to sounds in your abdomen using a stethoscope
- taps on your abdomen to check for pain and fullness or swelling

Dental Exam

For some people, a dental visit can be the first step toward discovering celiac disease. Dental enamel defects, such as white, yellow, or brown spots on the teeth, are a pretty common problem in people with celiac disease, especially children. These defects can help dentists and other healthcare professionals identify celiac disease.

Blood Tests

A healthcare professional may take a blood sample from you and send the sample to a lab to test for antibodies common in celiac disease. If blood test results are negative and your doctor still suspects celiac disease, he or she may order more blood tests.

Genetic Tests

If a biopsy and other blood tests do not clearly confirm celiac disease, your doctor may order genetic blood tests to check for certain gene changes, or variants. You are very unlikely to have celiac disease if these gene variants are not present. Having these variants alone is not enough to diagnose celiac disease because they also are common in people without the disease. In fact, most people with these genes will never get celiac disease.

Intestinal Biopsy

If blood tests suggest you have celiac disease, your doctor will perform a biopsy to be sure. During a biopsy, the doctor takes a small piece of tissue from your small intestine during a procedure called an upper gastrointestinal (GI) endoscopy.

Skin Biopsy

If a doctor suspects you have dermatitis herpetiformis, he or she will perform a skin biopsy. For a skin biopsy, the doctor removes tiny pieces of skin tissue to examine with a microscope.

A doctor examines the skin tissue and checks the tissue for antibodies common in celiac disease. If the skin tissue has the antibodies, a doctor will perform blood tests to confirm celiac

Do Doctors Screen For Celiac Disease?

Screening is testing for diseases when you have no symptoms. Doctors in the United States do not routinely screen people for celiac disease. However, blood relatives of people with celiac disease and those with type 1 diabetes should talk with their doctor about their chances of getting the disease.

Many researchers recommend routine screening of all family members, such as parents and siblings, for celiac disease. However, routine genetic screening for celiac disease is not usually helpful when diagnosing the disease.

disease. If the skin biopsy and blood tests both suggest celiac disease, you may not need an intestinal biopsy.

How Do Doctors Treat Celiac Disease?

A Gluten-Free Diet

Doctors treat celiac disease with a gluten-free diet. Gluten is a protein found naturally in wheat, barley, and rye that triggers a reaction if you have celiac disease. Symptoms greatly improve for most people with celiac disease who stick to a gluten-free diet. In recent years, grocery stores and restaurants have added many more gluten-free foods and products, making it easier to stay gluten free.

Your doctor may refer you to a dietitian who specializes in treating people with celiac disease. The dietitian will teach you how to avoid gluten while following a healthy diet. He or she will help you:

- check food and product labels for gluten

- design everyday meal plans

- make healthy choices about the types of foods to eat

For most people, following a gluten-free diet will heal damage in the small intestine and prevent more damage. You may see symptoms improve within days to weeks of starting the diet. The small intestine usually heals in 3 to 6 months in children. Complete healing can take several years in adults. Once the intestine heals, the villi, which were damaged by the disease, regrow and will absorb nutrients from food into the bloodstream normally.

An estimated 3 million people in the United States have celiac disease. In people with celiac disease, foods that contain gluten trigger production of antibodies that attack and damage the lining of the small intestine. Such damage limits the ability of celiac disease patients to absorb nutrients and puts them at risk of other very serious health problems, including nutritional deficiencies, osteoporosis, growth retardation, infertility, miscarriages, short stature, and intestinal cancers.

On August 2, 2013, U.S. Food and Drug Administration (FDA) issued a final rule defining "gluten-free" for food labeling, which will help consumers, especially those living with celiac disease, be confident that items labeled "gluten-free" meet a defined standard for gluten content.

(Source: "Gluten-Free Labeling Of Foods," U.S. Food and Drug Administration (FDA).)

Gluten-Free Diet And Dermatitis Herpetiformis

If you have dermatitis herpetiformis—an itchy, blistering skin rash—skin symptoms generally respond to a gluten-free diet. However, skin symptoms may return if you add gluten back into your diet. Medicines such as dapsone, taken by mouth, can control the skin symptoms. People who take dapsone need to have regular blood tests to check for side effects from the medicine.

Dapsone does not treat intestinal symptoms or damage, which is why you should stay on a gluten-free diet if you have the rash. Even when you follow a gluten-free diet, the rash may take months or even years to fully heal—and often comes back over the years.

Avoiding Medicines And Nonfood Products That May Contain Gluten

In addition to prescribing a gluten-free diet, your doctor will want you to avoid all hidden sources of gluten. If you have celiac disease, ask a pharmacist about ingredients in:

- herbal and nutritional supplements

- prescription and over-the-counter (OTC) medicines

- vitamin and mineral supplements

You also could take in or transfer from your hands to your mouth other products that contain gluten without knowing it. Products that may contain gluten include:

- children's modeling dough, such as Play-Doh

- cosmetics

- lipstick, lip gloss, and lip balm

- skin and hair products

- toothpaste and mouthwash

- communion wafers

Medications are rare sources of gluten. Even if gluten is present in a medicine, it is likely to be in such small quantities that it would not cause any symptoms.

Reading product labels can sometimes help you avoid gluten. Some product makers label their products as being gluten-free. If a product label doesn't list the product's ingredients, ask the maker of the product for an ingredients list.

What If Changing To A Gluten-Free Diet Isn't Working?

If you don't improve after starting a gluten-free diet, you may still be eating or using small amounts of gluten. You probably will start responding to the gluten-free diet once you find and cut out all hidden sources of gluten. Hidden sources of gluten include additives made with wheat, such as:

- modified food starch
- malt flavoring
- preservatives
- stabilizers

If you still have symptoms even after changing your diet, you may have other conditions or disorders that are more common with celiac disease, such as irritable bowel syndrome (IBS), lactose intolerance, microscopic colitis, dysfunction of the pancreas, and small intestinal bacterial overgrowth.

What Should I Avoid Eating If I Have Celiac Disease?

Avoiding foods with gluten, a protein found naturally in wheat, rye, and barley, is critical in treating celiac disease. Removing gluten from your diet will improve symptoms, heal damage to your small intestine, and prevent further damage over time. While you may need to avoid certain foods, the good news is that many healthy, gluten-free foods and products are available.

You should avoid all products that contain gluten, such as most cereal, grains, and pasta, and many processed foods. Be sure to always read food ingredient lists carefully to make sure the food you want to eat doesn't have gluten. In addition, discuss gluten-free food choices with a dietitian or healthcare professional who specializes in celiac disease.

What Should I Eat If I Have Celiac Disease?

Foods such as meat, fish, fruits, vegetables, rice, and potatoes without additives or seasonings do not contain gluten and are part of a well-balanced diet. You can eat gluten-free types of bread, pasta, and other foods that are now easier to find in stores, restaurants, and at special food companies. You also can eat potato, rice, soy, amaranth, quinoa, buckwheat, or bean flour instead of wheat flour.

In the past, doctors and dietitians advised against eating oats if you have celiac disease. Evidence suggests that most people with the disease can safely eat moderate amounts of oats, as long as they did not come in contact with wheat gluten during processing. You should talk with your healthcare team about whether to include oats in your diet.

When shopping and eating out, remember to:

- read food labels —especially on canned, frozen, and processed foods—for ingredients that contain gluten
- identify foods labeled "gluten-free"; by law, these foods must contain less than 20 parts per million, well below the threshold to cause problems in the great majority of patients with celiac disease
- ask restaurant servers and chefs about how they prepare the food and what is in it
- find out whether a gluten-free menu is available
- ask a dinner or party host about gluten-free options before attending a social gathering

Foods labeled gluten-free tend to cost more than the same foods that have gluten. You may find that naturally gluten-free foods are less expensive. With practice, looking for gluten can become second nature.

If you have just been diagnosed with celiac disease, you and your family members may find support groups helpful as you adjust to a new approach to eating.

Is A Gluten-Free Diet Safe If I Don't Have Celiac Disease?

In recent years, more people without celiac disease have adopted a gluten-free diet, believing that avoiding gluten is healthier or could help them lose weight. No current data suggests that the general public should maintain a gluten-free diet for weight loss or better health.

A gluten-free diet isn't always a healthy diet. For instance, a gluten-free diet may not provide enough of the nutrients, vitamins, and minerals the body needs, such as fiber, iron, and calcium. Some gluten-free products can be high in calories and sugar.

If you think you might have celiac disease, don't start avoiding gluten without first speaking with your doctor. If your doctor diagnoses you with celiac disease, he or she will put you on a gluten-free diet.

Gluten-Free Food Labeling Requirements

The U.S. Food and Drug Administration (FDA) published a rule defining what "gluten-free" means on food labels. The "gluten-free" for food labeling rule requires that any food with the terms "gluten-free," "no gluten," "free of gluten," and "without gluten" on the label must meet all of the definition's requirements.

While the FDA rule does not apply to foods regulated by the U.S. Department of Agriculture (USDA), including meat and egg products, it is often still observed.

Chapter 33

Scombrotoxin (Histamine) Poisoning

Scombrotoxin is a combination of substances, histamine prominent among them. Histamine is produced during decomposition of fish, when decarboxylase enzymes made by bacteria that inhabit (but do not sicken) the fish interact with the fish's naturally occurring histidine, resulting in histamine formation. Other vasoactive biogenic amines resulting from decomposition of the fish, such as putrescine and cadaverine, also are thought to be components of scombrotoxin. Time / temperature abuse of scombrotoxin-forming fish (e.g., tuna and mahi-mahi) create conditions that promote formation of the toxin. Scombrotoxin poisoning is closely linked to the accumulation of histamine in these fish.

FDA has established regulatory guidelines that consider fish containing histamine at 50 ppm or greater to be in a state of decomposition and fish containing histamine at 500 ppm or greater to be a public health hazard. The European Union issued Council Directive (91/493/EEC) in 1991, which states that when 9 samples taken from a lot of fish are analyzed for histamine, the mean value must not exceed 100 ppm; two samples may have a value of more than 100 ppm, but less than 200 ppm; and no sample may have a value exceeding 200 ppm.

Disease

The disease caused by scombrotoxin is called scombrotoxin poisoning or histamine poisoning. Treatment with antihistamine drugs is warranted when scombrotoxin poisoning is suspected.

- **Mortality:** No deaths have been confirmed to have resulted from scombrotoxin poisoning.

About This Chapter: This chapter includes text excerpted from "Bad Bug Book—Handbook Of Foodborne Pathogenic Microorganisms And Natural Toxins," U.S. Food and Drug Administration (FDA), October 24, 2017.

- **Dose:** In most cases, histamine levels in illness-causing (scombrotoxic) fish have exceeded 200 ppm, often above 500 ppm. However, there is some evidence that other biogenic amines also may play a role in the illness.

- **Onset:** The onset of intoxication symptoms is rapid, ranging from minutes to a few hours after consumption.

- **Disease/Complications:** Severe reactions (e.g., cardiac and respiratory complications) occur rarely, but people with pre-existing conditions may be susceptible. People on certain medications, including the antituberculosis drug isoniazid, are at increased risk for severe reactions.

- **Symptoms:** Symptoms of scombrotoxin poisoning include tingling or burning in or around the mouth or throat, rash or hives, drop in blood pressure, headache, dizziness, itching of the skin, nausea, vomiting, diarrhea, asthmatic-like constriction of air passage, heart palpitation, and respiratory distress.

- **Duration:** The duration of the illness is relatively short, with symptoms commonly lasting several hours, but, in some cases, adverse effects may persist for several days.

- **Route of entry:** Oral.

- **Pathway:** In humans, histamine exerts its effects on the cardiovascular system by causing blood-vessel dilation, which results in flushing, headache, and hypotension. It increases heart rate and contraction strength, leading to heart palpitations, and induces intestinal smooth-muscle contraction, causing abdominal cramps, vomiting, and diarrhea. Histamine also stimulates motor and sensory neurons, which may account for burning sensations and itching associated with scombrotoxin poisoning. Other biogenic amines, such as putrescine and cadaverine, may potentiate scombrotoxin poisoning by interfering with the enzymes necessary to metabolize histamine in the human body.

Frequency

Scombrotoxin poisoning is one of the most common forms of fish poisoning in the United States. From 1990 to 2007, outbreaks of scombrotoxin poisoning numbered 379 and involved 1,726 people, per reports to the Centers for Disease Control and Prevention (CDC). However, the actual number of outbreaks is believed to be far greater than that reported.

Sources

Fishery products that have been implicated in scombrotoxin poisoning include tuna, mahi-mahi, bluefish, sardines, mackerel, amberjack, anchovies, and others. Scombrotoxin-forming fish are commonly distributed as fresh, frozen, or processed products and may be consumed in a myriad of product forms. Distribution of the toxin within an individual fish or between cans in a case lot can be uneven, with some sections of a product capable of causing illnesses and others not.

Cooking, canning, and freezing do not reduce the toxic effects. Common sensory examination by the consumer cannot ensure the absence or presence of the toxin. Chemical analysis is a reliable test for evaluating a suspect fishery product. Histamine also may be produced in other foods, such as cheese and sauerkraut, which also has resulted in toxic effects in humans.

Diagnosis

Diagnosis of the illness is usually based on the patient's symptoms, time of onset, and the effect of treatment with antihistamine medication. The suspected food should be collected; rapidly chilled or, preferably, frozen; and transported to the appropriate laboratory for histamine analyses. Elevated levels of histamine in food suspected of causing scombrotoxin poisoning aid in confirming a diagnosis.

Target Populations

All humans are susceptible to scombrotoxin poisoning; however, as noted, the commonly mild symptoms can be more severe for individuals taking some medications, such as the anti-tuberculosis drug isoniazid. Because of the worldwide network for harvesting, processing, and distributing fishery products, the impact of the problem is not limited to specific geographic areas or consumption patterns.

Chapter 34

Sulfite Sensitivity

The U.S. Food and Drug Administration (FDA) has identified sulfites as one of the top-ten food allergens that affect one out of every 100 people living in the United States. Sulfites are used in food as preservatives to prevent discoloration or browning and to help deter spoilage. They are also used in the preparation, storage, and distribution of a wide variety of beverages. The wine industry, for example, has used sulfite as an ingredient for centuries, relying on its antioxidant and antibacterial properties to help keep wine fresh longer. During the 1970s and 1980s, the use of sulfites in food and beverages increased significantly, and in August 1986, the FDA banned the use of sulfites in fresh fruits and vegetables due to a growing number of cases of serious physical reactions to sulfites among many individuals.

In addition to their use as a food and beverage additive, sulfites are also commonly found in pharmaceutical products. These chemicals are often added to a number of medications, including those prescribed to treat asthma and allergic reactions, as a means of stabilizing and preserving the drugs for longer shelf life.

The exact causes of sulfite sensitivity are unclear; however, many experts believe there could be genetic or environmental factors involved. It also appears that individuals affected with asthma are particularly at risk for developing sulfite sensitivity. People often confuse sulfite sensitivity with an allergy; however, food allergies are usually caused by proteins in food, while the chemical sulfite does not contain proteins but is a salt of sulfurous acid.

About This Chapter: "Sulfite Sensitivity," © 2017 Omnigraphics. Reviewed November 2017; Text beginning with heading "Sulfite In Drug Products" is excerpted from "Food And Drug Administration Department Of Health And Human Services Subchapter C—Drugs: General," U.S. Food and Drug Administration (FDA), April 1, 2017.

Symptoms

The symptoms of sulfite sensitivity, which can range from mild to severe, take a minimum of 15 to 30 minutes to surface. They can include headache, hives, sneezing, sinus congestion, tightness of the throat, asthma attacks, runny nose, wheezing, shortness of breath, abdominal pain, nausea, coughing, skin inflammation, and skin rash.

Other health conditions that seem to have a link to sulfites include fibromyalgia, diabetes, depression, candida and other fungal infections, joint pain, immune deficiencies, skin conditions, irritable bowel syndrome (IBS), muscle weakness, nose bleeds, bloating, yeast infections, indigestion, heart palpitations, chronic fatigue syndrome, tooth pain, ear infections, and lethargy. In many cases, people can relieve some of these symptoms by maintaining a sulfite-free diet.

Asthma symptoms have been very closely linked to the intake of sulfites. Although these can vary from person to person, symptoms can range from mild wheezing to life-threatening asthma reactions. Consumption of food or beverages containing sulfite can trigger asthma attacks, but the inhalation of sulfur dioxide from foods containing sulfites may also cause asthmatic symptoms. In rare cases, sulfites have also been known to cause anaphylaxis, a severe, life-threating allergic reaction.

Diagnosis

In order to diagnose sulfite sensitivity, a healthcare provider will ask for a complete medical history, including a detailed description of symptoms. The healthcare provider may also ask about the patient's location when the symptoms occurred, as well as the type of food and beverages consumed. A doctor will conduct a thorough physical examination and will likely order lab work that might include blood tests and allergy skin tests.

For asthma attacks linked to sulfites, the healthcare provided may recommend a challenge procedure. This involves capsules or solutions of sulfites in increasing dosages over a period of two or more hours. Initially, a small dose of sulfite is administered to the sulfite-sensitive person. Mild doses are given to make sure only slight wheezing occurs and more severe reactions are avoided. But certain individuals who are sulfite-sensitive may not react to small doses, and in these cases a heavier dose may be required. If an asthmatic reaction takes place, then the lung function is measured, and the reaction is quickly reversed with the help of an inhaled bronchodilator medication.

Treatment

Avoidance is the best cure for sulfite sensitivity. Once a diagnosis is confirmed, a healthcare provider will determine a course of treatment. Many symptoms can be reduced or eliminated by avoiding foods, beverages, and medications that contain sulfites.

The following are some steps commonly recommended to address sulfite sensitivity:

- Knowing the names of sulfites and recognizing them on food labels.

- Avoiding foods that contain sulfite ingredients.

- Reading drug labels carefully, and consulting with a pharmacist for sulfite-free medications.

- If allergy seems to be severe, carrying a dose of epinephrine to treat severe reactions.

Certain medications might be prescribed by a healthcare provider to treat allergic reactions and other symptoms:

- Epinephrine for life-threatening allergic reactions.

- For asthma, an inhaler to help relieve airway inflammation.

- Antihistamines for swelling and itching.

- Corticosteroids for several swelling and itching.

Foods That May Contain Sulfites

Individuals with sulfite sensitivity need to educate themselves about foods that contain sulfites. Ingredients to look for on a food labels include sulfur dioxide, potassium bisulfite, sodium bisulfite, sodium metabisulfite, sodium sulfite, and potassium metabisulfite.

Some food items that may contain sulfite include maraschino cherries, all cheeses, wine vinegar, olives, pickles, and horseradish. Foods that contain gelatin, maple syrup, jams, jellies, and corn syrup can also have sulfites added to them, as can pizza, pie crust, tortillas, pasta, noodles, and crackers.

Alcoholic beverages, such as beer, wine, and mixed drinks, may contain sulfites to control or prevent fermentation, and beer and wine can also have natural sulfites in them. Sulfites might also be present in some nonalcoholic beverages, including fruit and vegetable juices and different kinds of tea.

Fish, meat, and other perishable food products require preservation until they are consumed, so many of them contain sulfites. For example, sulfites are used to help shellfish keep their color, preventing black spots on shrimp and lobster. They are added to meat to increase color so that the product looks fresher. Canned seafood, dried codfish, and seafood soups can contain sulfite, as can dried fruits and many other preserved products.

References

1. "Sulfite Sensitivity," Cleveland Clinic, December 30, 2016.

2. "Sulfite Allergies," Sulfites.org, n.d

3. "Health Library: Sulfite Sensitivity," Winchester Hospital, n.d.

4. "List of Foods for Sulfite Sensitivity," SFGate.com, n.d.

Sulfite In Drug Products

Sulfites are chemical substances that are added to certain drug products to inhibit the oxidation of the active drug ingredient. Oxidation of the active drug ingredient may result in instability and a loss of potency of the drug product. Examples of specific sulfites used to inhibit this oxidation process include sodium bisulfite, sodium metabisulfite, sodium sulfite, potassium bisulfite, and potassium metabisulfite. Recent studies have demonstrated that sulfites may cause allergic type reactions in certain susceptible persons, especially asthmatics. The labeling for any prescription drug product to which sulfites have been added as an inactive ingredient, regardless of the amount added, must bear the warning.

Labeling Requirement

The labeling required by 201.57 and 201.100(d) for prescription drugs for human use containing a sulfite, except epinephrine for injection when intended for use in allergic or other emergency situations, shall bear the warning statement "Contains (insert the name of the sulfite, e.g., sodium metabisulfite), a sulfite that may cause allergic-type reactions including anaphylactic symptoms and life-threatening or less severe asthmatic episodes in certain susceptible people. The overall prevalence of sulfite sensitivity in the general population is unknown and probably low. Sulfite sensitivity is seen more frequently in asthmatic than in nonasthmatic people." This statement shall appear in the "Warnings" section of the labeling.

The labeling required by 201.57 and 201.100(d) for sulfite-containing epinephrine for injection for use in allergic emergency situations shall bear the warning statement "Epinephrine is the preferred treatment for serious allergic or other emergency situations even though this product contains (insert the name of the sulfite, e.g., sodium metabisulfite), a sulfite that may in other products cause allergic type reactions including anaphylactic symptoms or life-threatening or less severe asthmatic episodes in certain susceptible persons. The alternatives to using epinephrine in a life-threatening situation may not be satisfactory. The presence of a sulfite(s) in this product should not deter administration of the drug for treatment of serious allergic or other emergency situations." This statement shall appear in the "Warnings" section of the labeling.

Is It Necessary To Declare Ingredients In Incidental Amounts? Can Sulfites Be Considered Incidental Additives?

The U.S. Food and Drug Administration (FDA) does not define "trace amounts"; however, there are some exemptions for declaring ingredients present in "incidental" amounts in a finished food. If an ingredient is present at an incidental level and has no functional or technical effect in the finished product, then it need not be declared on the label. An incidental additive is usually present because it is an ingredient of another ingredient. Note that major food allergens, regardless of whether they are present in the food in trace amounts, must be declared.

Sulfites added to any food or to any ingredient in any food and that has no technical effect in that food are considered to be incidental only if present at less than 10 ppm.

(Source: "Guidance For Industry: A Food Labeling Guide (6. Ingredient Lists)," U.S. Food and Drug Administration (FDA).)

Part Four
Other Common Allergy Triggers

Chapter 35

Pollen Allergies

> Each spring, summer, and fall, trees, weeds, and grasses release tiny pollen grains into the air. Some of the pollen ends up in your nose and throat. This can trigger a type of allergy called hay fever (also known as pollen allergy).
>
> *(Source: "Hay Fever," MedlinePlus, National Institutes of Health (NIH).)*

Ragweed Pollen

Ragweed and other weeds such as curly dock, lambs quarters, pigweed, plantain, sheep sorrel, and sagebrush are some of the most prolific producers of pollen allergens.

Although the ragweed pollen season runs from August to November, ragweed pollen levels usually peak in mid-September in many areas in the country.

In addition, pollen counts are highest between 5:00 a.m.–10:00 a.m. and on dry, hot, and windy days.

Preventive Strategies

- Avoid the outdoors between 5:00 a.m.–10:00 a.m. Save outside activities for late afternoon or after a heavy rain, when pollen levels are lower.

- Keep windows in your home and car closed to lower exposure to pollen. To keep cool, use air conditioners and avoid using window and attic fans.

About This Chapter: This chapter includes text excerpted from "Pollen," National Institute of Environmental Health Sciences (NIEHS), August 25, 2017.

- Be aware that pollen can also be transported indoors on people and pets.

- Dry your clothes in an automatic dryer rather than hanging them outside. Otherwise, pollen can collect on clothing and be carried indoors.

> Your healthcare provider may diagnose hay fever based on a physical exam and your symptoms. Sometimes skin or blood tests are used. Taking medicines and using nasal sprays can relieve symptoms. You can also rinse out your nose, but be sure to use distilled or sterilized water with saline. Allergy shots can help make you less sensitive to pollen and provide long-term relief.
>
> *(Source: "Hay Fever," MedlinePlus, National Institutes of Health (NIH).)*

Grass Pollen

As with tree pollen, grass pollen is regional as well as seasonal. In addition, grass pollen levels can be affected by temperature, time of day and rain.

Of the 1,200 species of grass that grow in North America, only a small percentage of these cause allergies. The most common grasses that can cause allergies are:

- Bermuda grass
- Johnson grass
- Kentucky bluegrass
- Orchard grass
- Sweet vernal grass
- Timothy grass

Preventive Strategies

- If you have a grass lawn, have someone else do the mowing. If you must mow the lawn yourself, wear a mask.

- Keep grass cut short.

- Choose ground covers that don't produce much pollen, such as Irish moss, bunch, and dichondra.

- Avoid the outdoors between 5:00 a.m.–10:00 a.m. Save outside activities for late afternoon or after a heavy rain, when pollen levels are lower.

- Keep windows in your home and car closed to lower exposure to pollen. To keep cool, use air conditioners and avoid using window and attic fans.

- Be aware that pollen can also be transported indoors on people and pets.

- Dry your clothes in an automatic dryer rather than hanging them outside. Otherwise, pollen can collect on clothing and be carried indoors.

Tree Pollen

Trees can aggravate your allergy whether or not they are on your property, since trees release large amounts of pollen that can be distributed miles away from the original source.

Trees are the earliest pollen producers, releasing their pollen as early as January in the Southern states and as late as May or June in the Northern states.

Most allergies are specific to one type of tree such as:

- catalpa
- elm
- hickory
- olive
- pecan
- sycamore
- walnut

or to the male cultivar of certain trees. The female of these species are totally pollen free:

- ash
- box elder
- cottonwood
- date palm
- maple (red)
- maple (silver)
- Phoenix palm

- poplar

- willow

Some people, though, do show cross reactivity among trees in the alder, beech, birch and oak family, and the juniper and cedar family.

Preventive Strategies

- If you buy trees for your yard, look for species that do not aggravate allergies such as crape myrtle, dogwood, fig, fir, palm, pear, plum, redbud and redwood trees or the female cultivars of ash, box elder, cottonwood, maple, palm, poplar or willow trees.

- Avoid the outdoors between 5:00 a.m.–10:00 a.m. Save outside activities for late afternoon or after a heavy rain, when pollen levels are lower.

- Keep windows in your home and car closed to lower exposure to pollen. To keep cool, use air conditioners and avoid using window and attic fans.

- Be aware that pollen can also be transported indoors on people and pets.

- Dry your clothes in an automatic dryer rather than hanging them outside. Otherwise, pollen can collect on clothing and be carried indoors.

Pollen allergy affects about 1 out of 10 Americans, according to the National Institute of Allergy and Infectious Diseases (NIAID). For some, symptoms can be controlled by using over-the-counter (OTC) medicine occasionally. Others have reactions that may more seriously disrupt the quality of their lives. Allergies can trigger or worsen asthma and lead to other health problems such as sinus infection (sinusitis) and ear infections in children.

(Source: "Itching For Allergy Relief?" U.S. Food and Drug Administration (FDA).)

Chapter 36

Pet Allergies

About Pets And Asthma

Proteins in your pet's skin flakes, urine, feces, saliva, and hair can trigger asthma. Dogs, cats, rodents (including hamsters and guinea pigs), and other warm-blooded mammals can trigger asthma in individuals with an allergy to animal dander.

The most effective method to control animal allergens in the home is to not allow animals in the home. If you remove an animal from the home, it is important to thoroughly clean the floors, walls, carpets, and upholstered furniture.

Some individuals may find isolation measures to be sufficiently effective. Isolation measures that have been suggested include keeping pets out of the sleeping areas, keeping pets away from upholstered furniture, carpets and stuffed toys, keeping the pet outdoors as much as possible and isolating sensitive individuals from the pet as much as possible.

What Is Pet Allergy?

Many people think animal allergies are caused by the fur or feathers of their pet. In fact, allergies are actually aggravated by:

- proteins secreted by oil glands and shed as dander

- proteins in saliva (which stick to fur when animals lick themselves)

About This Chapter: Text under the heading "About Pets And Asthma" is excerpted from "Asthma Triggers: Gain Control," U.S. Environmental Protection Agency (EPA), August 9, 2017; Text beginning with the heading "What Is Pet Allergy?" is excerpted from "Pets And Animals," National Institute of Environmental Health Sciences (NIEHS), April 20, 2017.

- aerosolized urine from rodents and guinea pigs

Keep in mind that you can sneeze with and without your pet being present. Although an animal may be out of sight, their allergens are not. This is because pet allergens are carried on very small particles. As a result, pet allergens can remain circulating in the air and remain on carpets and furniture for weeks and months after a pet is gone. Allergens may also be present in public buildings, schools, etc. where there are no pets.

Children exposed to high indoor levels of pet or pest allergens during infancy have a lower risk of developing asthma by 7 years of age, new research supported by the National Institutes of Health reveals. The findings, published September 19 in the *Journal of Allergy and Clinical Immunology*, may provide clues for the design of strategies to prevent asthma from developing.

Among 442 children for whom researchers had enough data to assess asthma status at age 7 years, 130 children (29 percent) had asthma. Higher concentrations of cockroach, mouse, and cat allergens present in dust samples collected from the children's homes during the first three years of life (at age 3 months, 2 years, and 3 years) were linked to a lower risk of asthma by age 7 years. The researchers observed a similar association for dog allergen, although it was not statistically significant, meaning it could be due to chance. Additional analysis indicated that exposure to higher levels of these four allergens at age 3 months was associated with a lower risk of developing asthma.

(Source: "Exposure To Pet And Pest Allergens During Infancy Linked To Reduced Asthma Risk," National Institutes of Health (NIH).)

Preventive Strategies

- Remove pets from your home if possible.

- If pet removal is not possible, keep them out of bedrooms and confined to areas without carpets or upholstered furniture.

- If possible, bathe pets weekly to reduce the amount of allergens.

- Wear a dust mask and gloves when near rodents.

- After playing with your pet, wash your hands and clean your clothes to remove pet allergens.

- Avoid contact with soiled litter cages.

- Dust often with a damp cloth.

The most effective method to control animal allergens in the home is to not allow animals in the home. If you remove an animal from the home, it is important to thoroughly clean the floors, walls, carpets, and upholstered furniture.

Some individuals may find isolation measures to be sufficiently effective. Isolation measures that have been suggested include keeping pets out of the sleeping areas, keeping pets away from upholstered furniture, carpets and stuffed toys, keeping the pet outdoors as much as possible and isolating sensitive individuals from the pet as much as possible.

(Source: "Asthma Triggers: Gain Control," U.S. Environmental Protection Agency (EPA).)

Chapter 37

Allergies And Other Health Effects Of Mold

What Are Molds?

Molds are fungi that can be found both indoors and outdoors. No one knows how many species of fungi exist but estimates range from tens of thousands to perhaps three hundred thousand or more. Molds grow best in warm, damp, and humid conditions, and spread and reproduce by making spores. Mold spores can survive harsh environmental conditions, such as dry conditions, that do not support normal mold growth.

What Are Some Of The Common Indoor Molds?

- Cladosporium
- Penicillium
- Alternaria
- Aspergillus

How Do Molds Affect People?

Some people are sensitive to molds. For these people, exposure to molds can cause symptoms such as nasal stuffiness, eye irritation, wheezing, or skin irritation. Some people, such as those with serious allergies to molds, may have more severe reactions. Severe reactions

About This Chapter: This chapter includes text excerpted from "Mold—Basic Facts," Centers for Disease Control and Prevention (CDC), September 26, 2017.

may occur among workers exposed to large amounts of molds in occupational settings, such as farmers working around moldy hay. Severe reactions may include fever and shortness of breath. Some people with chronic lung illnesses, such as obstructive lung disease, may develop mold infections in their lungs.

In 2004 the Institute of Medicine (IOM) found there was sufficient evidence to link indoor exposure to mold with upper respiratory tract symptoms, cough, and wheeze in otherwise healthy people; with asthma symptoms in people with asthma; and with hypersensitivity pneumonitis in individuals susceptible to that immune mediated condition. The IOM also found limited or suggestive evidence linking indoor mold exposure and respiratory illness in otherwise healthy children. In 2009, the World Health Organization (WHO) issued additional guidance, *The Guidelines for Indoor Air Quality: Dampness and Mould*.

Other studies have suggested a potential link of early mold exposure to development of asthma in some children, particularly among children who may be genetically susceptible to asthma development, and that selected interventions that improve housing conditions can reduce morbidity from asthma and respiratory allergies, but more research is needed in this regard.

Where Are Molds Found?

Molds are found in virtually every environment and can be detected, both indoors and outdoors, year round. Mold growth is encouraged by warm and humid conditions. Outdoors they can be found in shady, damp areas or places where leaves or other vegetation is decomposing. Indoors they can be found where humidity levels are high, such as basements or showers.

How Can People Decrease Mold Exposure?

Sensitive individuals should avoid areas that are likely to have mold, such as compost piles, cut grass, and wooded areas. Inside homes, mold growth can be slowed by controlling humidity levels and ventilating showers and cooking areas. If there is mold growth in your home, you should clean up the mold and fix the water problem. Mold growth can be removed from hard surfaces with commercial products, soap and water, or a bleach solution of no more than 1 cup of household laundry bleach in 1 gallon of water.

If you choose to use bleach to clean up mold:

- Never mix bleach with ammonia or other household cleaners. Mixing bleach with ammonia or other cleaning products will produce dangerous, toxic fumes.

- Open windows and doors to provide fresh air.

- Wear rubber boots, rubber gloves, and goggles during cleanup of affected area.

- If the area to be cleaned is more than 10 square feet, consult the U.S. Environmental Protection Agency (EPA) guide titled *Mold Remediation in Schools and Commercial Buildings*. Although focused on schools and commercial buildings, this document also applies to other building types.

- Always follow the manufacturer's instructions when using bleach or any other cleaning product.

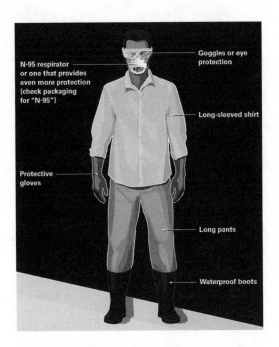

Figure 37.1. Protective Gears

(Source: "What To Wear Before Entering A Home Or Building With Mold Damage," Centers for Disease Control and Prevention (CDC).)

Specific Recommendations

- Keep humidity levels as low as you can—no higher than 50 percent—all day long. An air conditioner or dehumidifier will help you keep the level low. Bear in mind that humidity levels change over the course of a day with changes in the moisture in the air and the air temperature, so you will need to check the humidity levels more than once a day.

- Use an air conditioner or a dehumidifier during humid months.

- Be sure the home has adequate ventilation, including exhaust fans.

- Add mold inhibitors to paints before application.

- Clean bathrooms with mold killing products.

- Do not carpet bathrooms and basements.

- Remove or replace previously soaked carpets and upholstery.

If you are allergic to mold, or have asthma, being around mold may make your condition worse. If you have a chronic lung condition or a weak immune system, you could develop mold infections in your lungs and you should try to avoid buildings contaminated with mold.

Wear a protective mask, called an N95 respirator, when you clean up mold. You can buy N95s and half-face or full-face respirators at your local home supply store. Follow the instructions on the package to fit your respirator tightly on your face. A surgical mask or a bandanna will not prevent you from breathing in mold. See your healthcare provider if you think mold is making you sick.

(Source: "Dealing With Mold Allergies After A Disaster," Centers for Disease Control and Prevention (CDC).)

What Areas Have High Mold Exposures?

- Antique shops
- Greenhouses
- Saunas
- Farms
- Mills
- Construction areas
- Flower shops
- Summer cottages

I Found Mold Growing In My Home, How Do I Test The Mold?

Generally, it is not necessary to identify the species of mold growing in a residence, and the Centers for Disease Control and Prevention (CDC) does not recommend routine sampling for molds. Current evidence indicates that allergies are the type of diseases most often associated with molds. Since the susceptibility of individuals can vary greatly either because of the amount or type of mold, sampling and culturing are not reliable in determining your health risk. If you are susceptible to mold and mold is seen or smelled, there is a potential health risk; therefore, no matter what type of mold is present, you should arrange for its removal. Furthermore, reliable sampling for mold can be expensive, and standards for judging what is and what is not an acceptable or tolerable quantity of mold have not been established.

What Type Of Doctor Should I See Concerning Mold Exposure?

You should first consult a family or general healthcare provider who will decide whether you need referral to a specialist. Such specialists might include an allergist who treats patients with mold allergies or an infectious disease physician who treats mold infections. If an infection is in the lungs, a pulmonary physician might be recommended. Patients who have been exposed to molds in their workplace may be referred to an occupational physician.

My Landlord Or Builder Will Not Take Any Responsibility For Cleaning Up The Mold In My Home. Where Can I Go For Help?

If you feel your property owner, landlord, or builder has not been responsive to concerns you've expressed regarding mold exposure, you can contact your local board of health or housing authority. Applicable codes, insurance, inspection, legal, and similar issues about mold generally fall under state and local (not federal) jurisdiction. You could also review your lease or building contract and contact local or state government authorities, your insurance company, or an attorney to learn more about local codes and regulations and your legal rights. You can contact your county or state health department about mold issues in your area to learn about what mold assessment and remediation services they may offer.

I'm Sure That Mold In My Workplace Is Making Me Sick

If you believe you are ill because of exposure to mold in the building where you work, you should first consult your healthcare provider to determine the appropriate action to take to protect your health. Notify your employer and, if applicable, your union representative about your concern so that your employer can take action to clean up and prevent mold growth. To find out more about mold, remediation of mold, or workplace safety and health guidelines and regulations, you may also want to contact your local (city, county, or state) health department.

I Am Very Concerned About Mold In My Children's School And How It Affects Their Health.

If you believe your children are ill because of exposure to mold in their school, first consult their healthcare provider to determine the appropriate medical action to take. Contact the school's administration to express your concern and to ask that they remove the mold and prevent future mold growth. If needed, you could also contact the local school board.

Chapter 38

Cockroach Allergy

Cockroaches are one of the most common and allergenic of indoor pests. Some studies have found a strong association between the presence of cockroaches and increases in the severity of asthma symptoms in individuals who are sensitive to cockroach allergens.

These pests are common even in the cleanest of crowded urban areas and older dwellings. They are found in all types of neighborhoods.

The proteins found in cockroach saliva are particularly allergenic but the body and droppings of cockroaches also contain allergenic proteins.

Types Of Cockroaches

They range in size and color, and their shed skin contains allergens that can cause asthma. The most common cockroaches species include:

- German cockroach

- American cockroach

- Brownbanded cockroach

German Cockroach: *Blattella germanica*

German cockroaches are the most common cockroach found in the United States. The German cockroach is:

About This Chapter: Text in this chapter begins with excerpts from "Cockroaches," National Institute of Environmental Health Sciences (NIEHS), May 5, 2017; Text beginning with the heading "Types Of Cockroaches" is excerpted from "Managing Pests In Schools—Cockroaches And Schools," U.S. Environmental Protection Agency (EPA), May 24, 2017.

- 12 to 17mm (1/2 to 5/8 inch) long;

- tan to light brown; and

- has two dark brown stripes on the body region (pronotal shield) just behind the head.

Females will produce four to eight egg capsules during their lifetime, with each capsule containing approximately 40 eggs. The egg capsule is retained by the female until the eggs are ready to hatch, usually in 28 to 30 days.

German cockroaches are widespread and can be found in many indoor environments. Within these areas, the cockroaches prefer sites close to moisture and food, making them common pests in:

- Kitchens

- Bathrooms

- Food storage areas

American Cockroach: *Periplaneta americana*

The American cockroach is one of the largest cockroaches in the Northeast.

- It is about 40mm (1.5 inches) long with a reddish brown body.

- The center portion of the pronotal shield is light brown, while the outer edges are yellow.

Life Cycle: The female American cockroach will not retain the egg capsule for more than a day after its formation, instead dropping the capsule in some suitable site. Under some conditions it may be glued to a surface. The number of capsules produced by a female will range from 6 to 14, with each capsule containing 14 to 16 eggs. The eggs hatch in 50 to 55 days.

The American cockroach prefers dark, moist sites where it feeds on decaying organic matter. Such sites include:

- Basements

- Kitchens

- Clothes hampers

- Drains

- Bathroom plumbing or sewers

Brownbanded Cockroach: *Supella longipalpa*

The brownbanded cockroach is:

- 12 mm (1/2 inch) long;

- light brown; and

- has two lighter colored bands running across the body.

These bands are located at the base of the wings and on the abdomen. The bands are much darker during the immature stages.

Life Cycle: The brownbanded female carries the egg capsule for 24 to 48 hours before gluing it to a surface. The capsule contains approximately 18 eggs that hatch in 50–74 days. An adult female produces about 18 egg capsules over a lifespan of 10 months.

The brownbanded cockroach requires less moisture than other cockroaches. It is more prevalent in homes, apartments, hotels, and hospital rooms than in restaurants or stores. Evidence of this cockroach may be found:

- Behind pictures

- In furniture

- The underside of chairs and tables

- In upper kitchen cabinets

- On the upper shelves of closets and pantries

Health Concerns

Cockroaches can cause 2 potentially serious health problems. First, they may provoke allergic reactions. Second, they have been suggested as possible vectors of multidrug-resistant pathogens.

(Source: "Cockroaches (Ectobius vittiventris) In An Intensive Care Unit, Switzerland," Centers for Disease Control and Prevention (CDC).)

Cockroaches and their droppings may trigger an asthma attack. Their feces, saliva, eggs, and outer covering, or cuticles left behind on surfaces contain substances that are allergenic to humans, especially those with asthma or other respiratory conditions.

211

Within and on the surface of their bodies, cockroaches carry bacteria that can cause *salmonella*, *staphlylococcus*, and *streptococcus*, if deposited in food. Additionally, cockroach feces, skin sheddings and saliva can cause asthma and allergies, especially in children.

Cockroach Management Tips

To stay free of cockroach infestations:

- Don't allow dirty dishes to accumulate in the sink and remain there overnight.

- Keep food scraps in the refrigerator or in containers with tight-fitting lids.

- If small animals are in the classroom, keep the food in tightly sealed containers, and do not allow food to remain in the bowls overnight.

- Feed only what the animal will eat at the time of feeding.

- Remove garbage from the classroom and kitchen areas on a routine basis.

- Keep outside containers covered, especially at night.

- Periodically check and clean the evaporation pan under the refrigerator or freezer.

- Check the critical area between the stove and cabinet where grease and food scraps often accumulate.

- Pull the stove out periodically and clean thoroughly.

Preventive Strategies

- Keep food and garbage in closed, tight-lidded containers. Never leave food out in the kitchen.
- Do not leave out pet food or dirty food bowls.
- Eliminate water sources that attract these pests, such as leaky faucets and drain pipes.
- Mop the kitchen floor and wash countertops at least once a week.
- Plug up crevices around the house through which cockroaches can enter.
- Limit the spread of food around the house and especially keep food out of bedrooms.
- Use bait stations and other environmentally safe pesticides to reduce cockroach infestation.

(Source: "Cockroaches," National Institute of Environmental Health Sciences (NIEHS).)

Chapter 39

Dust Mites

Dust mites are tiny microscopic relatives of the spider and live on mattresses, bedding, upholstered furniture, carpets, and curtains.

These tiny creatures feed on the flakes of skin that people and pets shed daily and they thrive in warm and humid environments.

No matter how clean a home is, dust mites cannot be totally eliminated. However, the number of mites can be reduced by following the suggestions below.

Preventive Strategies

- Use a dehumidifier or air conditioner to maintain relative humidity at about 50 percent or below.

- Encase your mattress and pillows in dust-proof or allergen impermeable covers (available from specialty supply mail order companies, bedding and some department stores).

- Wash all bedding and blankets once a week in hot water (at least 130–140°F) to kill dust mites. Nonwashable bedding can be frozen overnight to kill dust mites.

- Replace wool or feathered bedding with synthetic materials and traditional stuffed animals with washable ones.

- If possible, replace wall-to-wall carpets in bedrooms with bare floors (linoleum, tile, or wood) and remove fabric curtains and upholstered furniture.

About This Chapter: Text in this chapter begins with excerpts from "Dust Mites," National Institute of Environmental Health Sciences (NIEHS), April 20, 2017; Text under the heading "Treating Dust Mite Allergy" is excerpted from "FDA Approves Odactra For House Dust Mite Allergies," U.S. Food and Drug Administration (FDA), March 1, 2017.

- Use a damp mop or rag to remove dust. Never use a dry cloth since this just stirs up mite allergens.

- Use a vacuum cleaner with either a double-layered microfilter bag or a high efficiency particulate air (HEPA) filter to trap allergens that pass through a vacuum's exhaust.

- Wear a mask while vacuuming to avoid inhaling allergens, and stay out of the vacuumed area for 20 minutes to allow any dust and allergens to settle after vacuuming.

Treating Dust Mite Allergy

The U.S. Food and Drug Administration (FDA) has approved Odactra, the first allergen extract to be administered under the tongue (sublingually) to treat house dust mite (HDM)-induced nasal inflammation (allergic rhinitis), with or without eye inflammation (conjunctivitis), in people 18 through 65 years of age.

"House dust mite allergic disease can negatively impact a person's quality of life," said Peter Marks, M.D., Ph.D., director of the FDA's Center for Biologics Evaluation and Research (CBER). "The approval of Odactra provides patients an alternative treatment to allergy shots to help address their symptoms."

House dust mite allergies are a reaction to tiny bugs that are commonly found in house dust. Dust mites, close relatives of ticks and spiders, are too small to be seen without a microscope. They are found in bedding, upholstered furniture, and carpeting. Individuals with house dust mite allergies may experience a cough, runny nose, nasal itching, nasal congestion, sneezing, and itchy and watery eyes.

Odactra exposes patients to house dust mite allergens, gradually training the immune system in order to reduce the frequency and severity of nasal and eye allergy symptoms. It is a once-daily tablet, taken year round, that rapidly dissolves after it is placed under the tongue. The first dose is taken under the supervision of a healthcare professional with experience in the diagnosis and treatment of allergic diseases. The patient is to be observed for at least 30 minutes for potential adverse reactions. Provided the first dose is well tolerated, patients can then take Odactra at home. It can take about eight to 14 weeks of daily dosing after initiation of Odactra for the patient to begin to experience a noticeable benefit.

The safety and efficacy of Odactra was evaluated in studies conducted in the United States, Canada, and Europe, involving approximately 2,500 people. Some participants received Odactra, while others received a placebo pill. Participants reported their symptoms and the need to use symptom-relieving allergy medications. During treatment, participants taking Odactra experienced a 16 to 18 percent reduction in symptoms and the need for additional medications compared to those who received a placebo.

The most commonly reported adverse reactions were nausea, itching in the ears and mouth, and swelling of the lips and tongue. The prescribing information includes a boxed warning that severe allergic reactions, some of which can be life threatening, can occur. As with other FDA-approved allergen extracts administered sublingually, patients receiving Odactra should be prescribed auto-injectable epinephrine.

Chapter 40

Smoking

Cigarette smoke contains a number of toxic chemicals and irritants. People with allergies may be more sensitive to cigarette smoke than others and research studies indicate that smoking may aggravate allergies.

Smoking does not just harm smokers but also those around them. Research has shown that children and spouses of smokers tend to have more respiratory infections and asthma than those of nonsmokers. In addition, exposure to secondhand smoke can increase the risk of allergic complications such as sinusitis and bronchitis.

Common symptoms of smoke irritation are burning or watery eyes, nasal congestion, coughing, hoarseness and shortness of breath presenting as a wheeze.

> Smokers are more likely than nonsmokers to develop heart disease, stroke, and lung cancer.
>
> Estimates show smoking increases the risk:
>
> - For coronary heart disease by 2 to 4 times
> - For stroke by 2 to 4 times
> - Of men developing lung cancer by 25 times
> - Of women developing lung cancer by 25.7 times
>
> Smoking causes diminished overall health, increased absenteeism from work, and increased healthcare utilization and cost.
>
> *(Sources: "Health Effects Of Cigarette Smoking," Centers for Disease Control and Prevention (CDC).)*

About This Chapter: This chapter includes text excerpted from "Cigarette Smoke," National Institute of Environmental Health Sciences (NIEHS), August 25, 2017.

217

Preventive Strategies

- Don't smoke and if you do, seek support to quit smoking.

- Seek smokefree environments in restaurants, theaters, and hotel rooms.

- Avoid smoking in closed areas like homes or cars where others may be exposed to secondhand smoke.

Make Your Home And Vehicles Smokefree For Cleaner Air And A Healthier Heart And Lungs

More than 58 million nonsmokers in the United States are still exposed to secondhand smoke, even though cigarette smoking rates are dropping and many states prohibit smoking in public places such as worksites, restaurants, and bars. In all, about 1 of every 4 nonsmokers is exposed to the dangerous chemicals in secondhand smoke.

Young children and African—Americans are more likely to be exposed to secondhand smoke than many other population groups.

- 2 in 5 children (aged 3 to 11 years), including 7 in 10 Black children (aged 3 to 11 years), are exposed, as are
- Nearly half of all Black nonsmokers.

Breathing secondhand smoke is also more common for renters and people at lower income levels, including:

- 2 in 5 people who live in poverty
- More than 1 in 3 people who live in rental housing

Secondhand smoke exposure occurs when nonsmokers breathe in tobacco smoke exhaled by smokers or when they breathe the smoke from burning tobacco products. The U.S. Environmental Protection Agency (EPA) has classified secondhand smoke as a Group A carcinogen—an agent that is known to cause cancer in humans—and the Surgeon General has concluded that there is no safe level of exposure to secondhand smoke.

Secondhand smoke contains dangerous chemicals that can damage the lungs and heart. It is known to cause heart disease and cancer in adult nonsmokers, and even brief exposure can trigger a heart attack or stroke. Secondhand smoke can also cause sudden infant death syndrome (SIDS), respiratory infections, ear infections, and asthma attacks in infants and children.

Every year, exposure to secondhand smoke causes:

- 41,000 adult nonsmokers to die from heart disease or lung cancer
- 400 infants to die from SIDS
- More than two and a half million nonsmokers have died from exposure to secondhand smoke since 1964

Smokefree Laws Save Lives, But Many Not Protected

In the last 25 years, 700 cities and 26 states plus the District of Columbia have passed comprehensive laws to protect nonsmokers by prohibiting smoking in indoor workplaces, restaurants, and bars. These local and state laws currently cover about half of the United States population and have helped reduce the number of people who are exposed to secondhand smoke.

In buildings without restrictions, smoke from common areas or other units where smoking occurs can seep into smokefree units!

Home Exposure Still A Problem

Even though more than 4 of every 5 households in the United States have adopted smokefree rules, secondhand smoke exposure in the home is still a serious problem. The home remains the major source of secondhand smoke exposure for children. The Surgeon General has indicated that making indoor spaces smokefree is the only way to provide nonsmokers with complete protection from secondhand smoke.

Limiting smoking to specific rooms, opening a window, or using air fresheners or fans is not enough to fully protect individuals in the home, including those who live in multiunit housing such as apartments, condos, and government funded housing. Many people who live in public housing are especially affected by secondhand smoke, including the elderly, children, and people with disabilities. A few cities have passed laws restricting smoking in multiunit housing and several hundred housing authorities have adopted smokefree policies. However, in buildings without restrictions, smoke from common areas or other units where smoking occurs can seep into smokefree units.

What's The Solution?

There are many ways to protect people from secondhand smoke exposure.

- **Parents** can ensure their homes and vehicles are smokefree and keep their children away from public places where smoking is allowed.

- **Housing authorities and landlords** can make their properties—especially multiunit buildings—smokefree to protect the health of all residents. For example, all 20 public housing authorities in Maine have made their buildings smokefree.

- **Cities and states** can pass smokefree laws to protect nonsmokers in all indoor workplaces, restaurants, bars, and casinos, and can work to increase availability of smokefree multiunit housing. In California, 15 counties and cities have passed ordinances restricting smoking in multiunit housing.

By working together, individuals and communities can eliminate the serious health hazards for nonsmokers that can result from exposure to secondhand smoke.

Chapter 41

Sting Allergies

Warm weather makes it easier to spend more time outdoors, but it also brings out the bugs. Ticks are usually harmless. But a tick bite can lead to Lyme disease, which is caused by the bacterium Borrelia burgdorferi. The bacteria are transmitted to people by the black-legged deer tick, which is about the size of a pinhead and usually lives on deer. Infected ticks can also cause other diseases, such as Rocky Mountain spotted fever.

Another insect-borne illness, West Nile virus, is transmitted by infected mosquitoes and usually produces mild symptoms in healthy people. But the illness can be serious for older people and those with compromised immune systems.

Most reactions to bees and other stinging insects are mild, but severe allergic reactions can be deadly. An allergic reaction can occur even if a person has been stung before with no complications.

Symptoms of a scorpion sting may include:

- A stinging or burning sensation at the injection site (very little swelling or inflammation)
- Positive "tap test" (i.e., extreme pain when the sting site is tapped with a finger)
- Restlessness
- Convulsions
- Roving eyes

About This Chapter: This chapter includes text excerpted from "Beware Of Bug Bites And Stings," U.S. Food and Drug Administration (FDA), August 24, 2017.

- Staggering gait
- Thick tongue sensation
- Slurred speech
- Drooling
- Muscle twitches
- Abdominal pain and cramps
- Respiratory depression

These symptoms usually subside within 48 hours, although stings from a bark scorpion can be life threatening.

(Source: "Insects And Scorpions," Centers for Disease Control and Prevention (CDC).)

What Can I Do To Keep Insects Away?

- Use structural barriers such as window screens and netting.

- Avoid wooded, brushy, and grassy areas when possible.

- Don't wear heavily scented soaps and perfumes.

- Use caution eating outside and drinking; don't leave drinks and garbage cans uncovered.

- Don't wear bright colors, which attract bees.

- Wear long sleeves and long pants when possible.

- Tuck pant legs into socks or shoes.

- Wear a hat for extra protection.

- Get rid of containers with standing water that give mosquitoes a breeding ground. Examples include water in flowerpots and outdoor pet dishes.

- Use insect repellent if nonchemical methods are ineffective and you spend time in tall grass and woody areas.

- Treat camping gear, clothes, and shoes with permethrin, which repels and kills ticks, mosquitoes, and other insects. Clothing that is pretreated with permethrin is also commercially available.

What's The Proper Way To Use Insect Repellent?

It's okay to use insect repellent and sunscreen at the same time. The general recommendation is to apply sunscreen first, followed by repellent. There are also some combination products that contain both insect repellent and sunscreen. U.S. Food and Drug Administration (FDA) regulates sunscreen as an over-the-counter (OTC) drug. The U.S. Environmental Protection Agency (EPA) regulates insect repellent products.

- Use insect repellent that contains active ingredients that have been registered with EPA. An EPA registration number on the product label means the product has been evaluated by EPA to ensure that it will not pose unreasonable harmful effects on people and the environment.

- Spray insect repellent on clothes or skin, but not on the face.

- Don't use insect repellent on babies. Repellent used on older children should contain no more than 10 percent DEET (N,N-Diethyl-meta-toluamide). Oil of eucalyptus products should not be used in children under 3 years.

- Don't use insect repellent that's meant for people on your pets.

- Use insect repellent according to the labeled instructions.

- Avoid applying it to children's hands, around the eyes, or to areas where there are cuts and irritated skin.

- Store insect repellent out of children's reach.

- Wash the repellent off with soap and water and contact a Poison Control Center (800-222-1222) if you experience a reaction to insect repellent.

- After returning indoors, wash skin with soap and water to remove repellent.

What's The Best Way To Remove A Bee Stinger?

It's best to scrape a stinger away in a side-to-side motion with a straight-edged object like a credit card. Don't use tweezers because it may push more venom into the skin. After removing a stinger, wash the area with soap and water. You can apply ice or another cold compress to help reduce swelling.

What Should I Do If I Find A Tick On Me Or My Child?

Wearing light-colored clothing makes it easier to spot ticks. Check for ticks after outdoor activities. If you find a tick, remove it with tweezers. Grasp the tick as close to the skin as possible and pull it straight out. Then drop it in a plastic bag, seal it up, and throw it away. Early removal of a tick is important because a tick generally has to be on the skin for 36 hours to transmit Lyme disease. People who want to get a tick tested for disease or other information could check with their local health departments to see if they offer tick testing. After removing a tick, you can cleanse the area of the tick bite with antiseptic, such as rubbing alcohol or soap and water.

What Can Be Done For Itching And Pain From Bites And Stings?

Oral OTC antihistamines can bring itch relief. Oral OTC drugs, such as ibuprofen and acetaminophen, can provide relief of pain from bites and stings.

In addition, there are many topical OTC drugs that are applied to the skin and can provide itch and pain relief. Some of these topical OTC drugs are labeled as "external analgesics" or "topical analgesics." They contain ingredients such as hydrocortisone, pramoxine, and lidocaine. There are also topical OTC drugs labeled as "skin protectants" that provide itch relief for insect bites and stings. These products contain ingredients such as colloidal oatmeal and sodium bicarbonate.

Keep kids' nails short. If they scratch the area and break the skin, it can lead to a bacterial infection that will require treatment with antibiotics.

When Is Medical Attention Needed?

Most bites and stings are minor and can be treated at home. But you should seek medical attention if you experience the following symptoms:

- **Signs of allergic reaction:** Some people can experience anaphylaxis, a severe, life-threatening allergic reaction. This is a medical emergency that warrants calling 9-1-1 immediately. Signs of an allergic reaction, which may occur within seconds to minutes, include sneezing, wheezing, hives, nausea, vomiting, diarrhea, sudden anxiety, dizziness, difficulty breathing, chest tightness, and itching or swelling of the eyes, lips, or other areas of the face. If you or your child has ever had an allergic reaction to a sting or bite, you should be evaluated by an allergist. In some cases, you may be advised to wear a medical identification tag that states the allergy, and to carry epinephrine, a medication used to treat serious or life-threatening allergic reactions. Sometimes allergy shots may also be recommended.

- **Symptoms of Lyme disease:** Lyme disease, which is transmitted through the bite of an infected tick, can cause fever, headaches, fatigue, and a skin rash that looks like a circular red patch, or "bull's-eye." Left untreated, infection can spread to the joints, heart, and nervous system. It is rarely, if ever, fatal. Patients who are treated with antibiotics in the early stages of the infection usually recover rapidly and completely. Antibiotics commonly used for oral treatment include doxycycline, amoxicillin, or cefuroxime axetil (Ceftin). People with certain illnesses related to the heart or the nervous system require intravenous treatment with drugs such as ceftriaxone or penicillin.

- **Symptoms of West Nile virus:** West Nile virus, which is transmitted by infected mosquitoes, can produce flu-like symptoms including fever, headache, body aches, and skin rash. While most infected individuals have mild disease and recover spontaneously, infection can be serious or even fatal. There is no specific treatment for West Nile virus.

- **Symptoms of Rocky Mountain spotted fever:** Initial symptoms may include fever, nausea, vomiting, severe headache, muscle pain, and lack of appetite. The characteristic red, spotted rash of Rocky Mountain spotted fever is usually not seen until the sixth day or later after symptoms begin. But as many as 10 percent to 15 percent of patients may never develop a rash. Rocky Mountain spotted fever is treated with antibiotics.

- **Signs of infection:** It is normal for a bite or sting to result in redness of the affected area and minor swelling. But if a bite or sting becomes infected, a fever may develop or the redness or soreness may worsen. In cases of infection, an antibiotic is the typical treatment.

Chapter 42

Nickel Allergy

What Is Nickel?

Pure nickel is a hard, silvery white metal, which has properties that make it very desirable for combining with other metals to form mixtures called alloys. Some of the metals that nickel can be alloyed with are iron, copper, chromium, and zinc. These alloys are used in making metal coins and jewelry and in industry for making items such as valves and heat exchangers. Most nickel is used to make stainless steel. There are also compounds consisting of nickel combined with many other elements, including chlorine, sulfur, and oxygen. Many of these nickel compounds are water soluble (dissolve fairly easily in water) and have a characteristic green color. Nickel and its compounds have no characteristic odor or taste. Nickel compounds are used for nickel plating, to color ceramics, to make some batteries, and as substances known as catalysts that increase the rate of chemical reactions.

Nickel combined with other elements occurs naturally in the earth's crust. It is found in all soil, and is also emitted from volcanoes. Nickel is the 24th most abundant element. In the environment, it is primarily found combined with oxygen or sulfur as oxides or sulfides. Nickel is also found in meteorites and on the ocean floor in lumps of minerals called sea floor nodules. The earth's core is composed of 6 percent nickel. Nickel is released into the atmosphere during nickel mining and by industries that make or use nickel, nickel alloys, or nickel compounds. These industries also might discharge nickel in wastewater. Nickel is also released into the atmosphere by oil burning power plants, coal burning power plants, and trash incinerators.

About This Chapter: This chapter includes text excerpted from "Toxic Substances Portal—Nickel," Agency for Toxic Substances and Disease Registry (ATSDR), Centers for Disease Control and Prevention (CDC), January 21, 2015.

There are no nickel mining operations in the United States. Much of our nickel used in industries comes from recycling nickel containing alloys or is imported mainly from Canada and Russia.

What Happens To Nickel When It Enters The Environment?

Nickel may be released to the environment from the stacks of large furnaces used to make alloys or from power plants and trash incinerators. The nickel that comes out of the stacks of power plants attaches to small particles of dust that settle to the ground or are taken out of the air in rain or snow. It usually takes many days for nickel to be removed from the air. If the nickel is attached to very small particles, it can take more than a month to settle out of the air. Nickel can also be released in industrial wastewater. A lot of nickel released into the environment ends up in soil or sediment where it strongly attaches to particles containing iron or manganese. Under acidic conditions, nickel is more mobile in soil and might seep into groundwater. Nickel does not appear to concentrate in fish. Studies show that some plants can take up and accumulate nickel. However, it has been shown that nickel does not accumulate in small animals living on land that has been treated with nickel containing sludge.

How Might I Be Exposed To Nickel?

Nickel normally occurs at very low levels in the environment, so very sensitive methods are needed to detect nickel in most environmental samples. Food is the major source of exposure to nickel. You may also be exposed to nickel by breathing air, drinking water, or smoking tobacco containing nickel. Skin contact with soil, bath or shower water, or metals containing nickel, as well as, metals plated with nickel can also result in exposure. Stainless steel and coins contain nickel. Some jewelry is plated with nickel or made from nickel alloys. Patients may be exposed to nickel in artificial body parts made from nickel containing alloys. Exposure of an unborn child to nickel is through the transfer of nickel from the mother's blood to fetal blood. Likewise, nursing infants are exposed to nickel through the transfer of nickel from the mother to breast milk. However, the concentration of nickel in breast milk is either similar or less than the concentration of nickel in infant formulas and cow's milk.

The exact form of nickel we are exposed to, including at most hazardous waste sites, is often not known. Much of the nickel found in air, soil, sediment, and rock is so strongly attached to dust and soil particles or embedded in minerals that it is not readily taken up by plants and animals and therefore cannot easily affect your health. In water and wastewater, nickel can exist either dissolved in water or attached to material suspended in water.

The concentration of nickel in the water of rivers and lakes is very low, with the average concentration usually less than 10 parts of nickel in a billion parts of water (ppb). The level of nickel in water is often so low that it cannot be measured unless very sensitive instruments are used. The average concentration of nickel in drinking water in the United States is between 2 and 4.3 ppb. However, you may be exposed to higher than average levels of nickel in drinking water if you live near industries that process or use nickel. The highest levels of nickel in drinking water, about 72 ppb, were found near areas of a large natural nickel deposit where nickel is mined and refined.

Soil usually contains between 4 and 80 parts of nickel in a million parts of soil (ppm; 1 ppm=1,000 ppb). The highest soil concentrations (up to 9,000 ppm) are found near industries that extract nickel from ore. High concentrations of nickel occur as dust that is released into air from stacks during processing and settles on the ground. You may be exposed to nickel in soil by skin contact. Children may also be exposed to nickel by eating soil.

Food contains nickel and is the major source of nickel exposure for the general population. You eat about 170 micrograms of nickel in your food every day. Foods naturally high in nickel include chocolate, soybeans, nuts, and oatmeal. Our daily intake of nickel from drinking water is only about 2 micrograms. We breathe in between 0.1 and 1 micrograms nickel/day, excluding nickel in tobacco smoke. We are exposed to nickel when we handle coins and touch other metals containing nickel.

You may be exposed to higher levels of nickel if you work in industries that process or use nickel. You also may be exposed to nickel by breathing dust or fumes (as from welding) or by skin contact with nickel containing metal and dust or solutions containing dissolved nickel compounds.

How Can Nickel Enter And Leave My Body?

Nickel can enter your body when you breathe air containing nickel, when you drink water or eat food that contains nickel, and when your skin comes into contact with nickel. If you breathe air that contains nickel, the amount of nickel you inhale that reaches your lungs and enters your blood depends on the size of the nickel particles. If the particles are large, they stay in your nose. If the particles are small, they can enter deep into your lungs.

More nickel is absorbed from your lungs into your body when the nickel particles can dissolve easily in water. When the particles do not dissolve easily in water, the nickel may remain in your lungs for a long time. Some of these nickel particles can leave the lungs with mucus that you spit out or swallow. More nickel will pass into your body through your stomach and intestines if you drink water containing nickel than if you eat food containing the same amount of nickel.

A small amount of nickel can enter your bloodstream from skin contact. After nickel gets into your body, it can go to all organs, but it mainly goes to the kidneys. The nickel that gets into your bloodstream leaves in the urine. After nickel is eaten, most of it leaves quickly in the feces, and the small amount that gets into your blood leaves in the urine.

How Can Nickel Affect My Health?

Scientists use many tests to protect the public from harmful effects of toxic chemicals and to find ways for treating persons who have been harmed.

One way to learn whether a chemical will harm people is to determine how the body absorbs, uses, and releases the chemical. For some chemicals, animal testing may be necessary. Animal testing may also help identify health effects such as cancer or birth defects. Without laboratory animals, scientists would lose a basic method for getting information needed to make wise decisions that protect public health. Scientists have the responsibility to treat research animals with care and compassion. Scientists must comply with strict animal care guidelines because laws today protect the welfare of research animals.

The most common harmful health effect of nickel in humans is an allergic reaction. Approximately 10–20 percent of the population is sensitive to nickel. A person can become sensitive to nickel when jewelry or other items containing nickel are in direct contact and prolonged contact with the skin. Wearing jewelry containing nickel in ears or other body parts that have been newly pierced may also sensitize a person to nickel. However, not all jewelry containing nickel releases enough of the nickel ion to sensitize a person. Once a person is sensitized to nickel, further contact with the metal may produce a reaction. The most common reaction is a skin rash at the site of contact. In some sensitized people, dermatitis (a type of skin rash) may develop in an area of the skin that is away from the site of contact. For example, hand eczema (another type of skin rash) is fairly common among people sensitized to nickel. Some workers exposed to nickel by inhalation can become sensitized and have asthma attacks, but this is rare.

People who are sensitive to nickel have reactions when nickel comes into prolonged contact with the skin. Some sensitized individuals react when they eat nickel in food or water or breathe dust containing nickel. More women are sensitive to nickel than men. This difference between men and women is thought to be a result of greater exposure of women to nickel through jewelry and other metal items.

People who are not sensitive to nickel must eat very large amounts of nickel to suffer harmful health effects. Workers who accidentally drank light green water containing 250 ppm of nickel from a contaminated drinking fountain had stomach aches and suffered adverse effects in their blood (increased red blood cells) and kidneys (increased protein in the urine). This concentration of nickel is more than 100,000 times greater than the amount usually found in drinking water.

The most serious harmful health effects from exposure to nickel, such as chronic bronchitis, reduced lung function, and cancer of the lung and nasal sinus, have occurred in people who have breathed dust containing certain nickel compounds while working in nickel refineries or nickel processing plants.

Exposure to high levels of nickel compounds that dissolve easily in water (soluble) may also result in cancer when nickel compounds that are hard to dissolve (less soluble) are present, or when other chemicals that can produce cancer are present. The concentrations of soluble and less-soluble nickel compounds that were found to have produced cancers were 100,000 to 1 million times greater than the usual level of nickel in the air in the United States. The U.S. Department of Health and Human Services (DHHS) has determined that nickel metal may reasonably be anticipated to be a carcinogen and nickel compounds are known human carcinogens. The International Agency for Research on Cancer (IARC) has determined that some nickel compounds are carcinogenic to humans and that metallic nickel may possibly be carcinogenic to humans. The EPA has determined that nickel refinery dust and nickel subsulfide are human carcinogens. These cancer classifications were based on studies of nickel workers and laboratory animals.

Lung inflammation and damage to the nasal cavity have been observed in animals exposed to nickel compounds. At high concentrations, the lung damage is severe enough to affect lung function. Long-term exposure to lower levels of a nickel compound that dissolves easily in water did not produce cancer in animals. Lung cancer developed in rats exposed for a long time to nickel compounds that do not dissolve easily in water.

Oral exposure of humans to high levels of soluble nickel compounds through the environment is extremely unlikely. Because humans have only rarely been exposed to high levels of nickel in water or food, much of the knowledge of the harmful effects of nickel is based on animal studies. Eating or drinking levels of nickel much greater than the levels normally found in food and water have been reported to produce lung disease in dogs and rats and to affect the stomach, blood, liver, kidneys, and immune system in rats and mice, as well as their reproduction and development.

How Can Nickel Affect Children?

The potential health effects in humans from exposures during the period from conception to maturity at 18 years of age.

It is likely that the health effects seen in children exposed to nickel will be similar to the effects seen in adults. It's not clearly known whether children differ from adults in their susceptibility to nickel. Human studies that examined whether nickel can harm the developing fetus are inconclusive. Animal studies have found increases in newborn deaths and decreases in newborn weight after ingesting nickel.

These doses are 1,000 times higher than levels typically found in drinking water. It is likely that nickel can be transferred from the mother to an infant in breast milk and can cross the placenta. The nickel levels in breast milk are likely to be similar to the levels in cow's milk based or soy milk based infant formula

---

How Can Families Reduce The Risk Of Exposure To Nickel?

If your doctor finds that you have been exposed to substantial amounts of nickel, ask whether your children might also have been exposed. Your doctor might need to ask your state health department to investigate.

People may be exposed to nickel by wearing jewelry that contains nickel. In some people, wearing jewelry that contains nickel produces skin irritation. Avoiding jewelry containing nickel will eliminate risks of exposure to this source of this metal.

Other sources of nickel exposure are through foods that you eat and drinking water. However, the amount of nickel in foods and drinking water are too low to be of concern.

Is There A Medical Test To Determine Whether I Have Been Exposed To Nickel?

Measurements of the amount of nickel in your blood, feces, and urine can be used to estimate your exposure to nickel. More nickel was found in the urine of workers who were exposed to nickel compounds that dissolve easily in water (soluble) than in the urine of workers exposed to compounds that are hard to dissolve (less soluble). This means that it is easier to tell if you have been exposed to soluble nickel compounds than less soluble compounds. The nickel measurements do not accurately predict potential health effects from exposure to nickel.

What Recommendations Has The Federal Government Made To Protect Human Health?

The federal government develops regulations and recommendations to protect public health. Regulations can be enforced by law. The EPA, the Occupational Safety and Health Administration (OSHA), and the U.S. Food and Drug Administration (FDA) are some federal agencies that develop regulations for toxic substances. Recommendations provide valuable guidelines to protect public health, but cannot be enforced by law. The Agency for Toxic Substances and Disease Registry (ATSDR) and the National Institute for Occupational Safety and Health (NIOSH) are two federal organizations that develop recommendations for toxic substances.

Regulations and recommendations can be expressed as "not-to-exceed" levels, that is, levels of a toxic substance in air, water, soil, or food that do not exceed a critical value that is usually based on levels that affect animals; they are then adjusted to levels that will help protect humans. Sometimes these not-to-exceed levels differ among federal organizations because they used different exposure times (an 8-hour workday or a 24-hour day), different animal studies, or other factors. Recommendations and regulations are also updated periodically as more information becomes available.

Chapter 43

Hair Dye Allergy

The U.S. Food and Drug Administration (FDA) often receives questions about the safety and regulation of hair dyes. Most of these products belong to a category called "coal tar" hair dyes.

Color additives, with the exception of coal tar hair dyes, need FDA approval before they're permitted for use in cosmetics.

FDA's ability to take action against coal tar hair dyes associated with safety concerns is limited by law. It's important to follow the directions on the label. It is also important to be an informed consumer and understand the risks.

What Are Coal Tar Hair Dyes?

The term "coal tar colors" dates back to the time when these coloring materials were by-products of the coal industry. Today, most are made from petroleum, but the original name is still used. Coal tar hair dyes—those coal tar colors used for dyeing hair—include permanent, semipermanent, and temporary hair dyes.

Coal tar colors are also called "synthetic organic" colors. That's because, to a chemist, a "synthetic" compound is one formed from simpler compounds and an "organic" compound is one that contains carbon atoms.

About This Chapter: This chapter includes text excerpted from "Cosmetics—Hair Dyes," U.S. Food and Drug Administration (FDA), August 25, 2015.

What The Law Says About Coal Tar Hair Dyes

Under the Federal Food, Drug, and Cosmetic Act (FD and C Act), a law passed by Congress, color additives must be approved by FDA for their intended use before they are used in FDA regulated products, including cosmetics. Other cosmetic ingredients do not need FDA approval. FDA can take action against a cosmetic on the market if it is harmful to consumers when used in the customary or expected way and used according to labeled directions.

How the law treats coal tar hair dyes:

- FDA cannot take action against a coal tar hair dye, as long as the label includes a special caution statement and the product comes with adequate directions for consumers to do a skin test before they dye their hair. This is the caution statement:

  Caution: This product contains ingredients which may cause skin irritation on certain individuals and a preliminary test according to accompanying directions should first be made. This product must not be used for dyeing the eyelashes or eyebrows; to do so may cause blindness. (FD and C Act, 601(a))

- Coal tar hair dyes, unlike color additives in general, do not need FDA approval. (FD and C Act, 601(e)).

But there are limits to this exception:

- FDA may take action if a harmful coal tar hair dye product if—

- it does not have the caution statement on its label or come with adequate directions for a skin test, or

- an ingredient other than the coal tar hair dye itself is harmful.

- "Coal tar hair dyes" are not eyebrow or eyelash dyes. Color additives intended for dyeing the eyebrows or eyelashes need FDA approval for that use. No color additives are approved for dyeing the eyebrows or eyelashes.

Safety Issues

While many people use coal tar hair dyes, FDA is aware of the following problems:

Eye injuries: Hair dyes have caused eye injuries, including blindness, when used in the eye area. Eyebrow and eyelash dyeing are not permitted uses of coal tar hair dyes.

Allergic reactions: Some coal tar hair dyes can cause allergic reactions or sensitization that may result in skin irritation and hair loss. People can develop sensitivities with repeated exposure. In addition, formulations may change over time. So, it's possible to have a reaction even if you have dyed your hair in the past, without a problem. That's why it's important to follow the instructions and do the skin test before every use. Even if you don't see a reaction to the skin test, it's still possible to have a reaction when you dye your hair.

One hair dye ingredient, p-phenylenediamine, or "PPD," has been implicated more prominently in leading to allergic reactions. Some people may become allergic to PPD from other exposures, including occupational exposures. This is called "cross sensitization." Here are some examples;

- Some temporary tattoo inks, sometimes marketed as "black henna"
- Certain textile dyes, ballpoint pen inks, some color additives used in foods and drugs, and other dyes used in semi permanent and temporary hair dyes
- Rubber and other latex products
- Benzocaine and procaine, local anesthetics used by doctors and dentists
- Para-aminosalicylic acid, a drug used to treat tuberculosis
- Sulfonamides, sulfones, and sulfa drugs
- Para-aminobenzoic acid (PABA) disclaimer icon, a naturally occurring compound used in some sunscreens disclaimer icon and in some cosmetics.

Temporary tattoo artists who use coal tar hair dyes to color people's skin are misusing these products and ingredients, because coal tar hair dyes are not intended to be used for staining the skin. While FDA regulates cosmetics products on the market, professional practice is generally subject to state and local authorities, not FDA.

If you have a reaction to a hair dye or tattoo, ask your healthcare provider about treatment. If you know what ingredient caused the problem, you may be able to find a product that doesn't contain that ingredient. If you color your hair yourself, check the list of ingredients on the label for any you wish to avoid. If you have your hair colored at a salon, your stylist may be able to tell you the ingredients, or you may wish to check with the manufacturer.

Other Types Of Hair Coloring Products

- Hair coloring materials made from plant or mineral sources are regulated the same as other color additives. They must be approved by FDA and listed in the color additive regulations.

Color additives approved for use on hair include henna (from the Lawsonia plant) as well as lead acetate and bismuth citrate, both of which are used in "progressive" hair dyes that darken hair gradually with repeated applications. Of note, temporary tattoos marketed as "black henna" contain PPD and may increase your risk of allergy to hair dyes. Hair dyes are not meant to be used for staining your skin.

Unusual Colors

People sometime ask whether unusual colors such as pink, orange, blue, and green are regulated differently from other hair dyes. How a hair dye is regulated depends on whether it is a coal-tar hair dye or is made from plant or mineral materials, not on the shade.

Do a patch test on your skin every time before dyeing your hair. Put a small amount of dye on a quarter-sized area of skin in the bend of your elbow. Leave it there for 48 hours. If you get a rash, do not use the dye.

P-phenylene diamine (PPD) is a common hair dye ingredient that some people become allergic to. If you want to avoid PPD, check the ingredient list on the hair dye label. In addition, if you are avoiding PPD, don't get "black henna" tattoos, which are also likely to contain that ingredient.

(Source: "Hair Dyes And Relaxers: Safety Tips," U.S. Food and Drug Administration (FDA).)

Coal Tar Hair Dye Safety Checklist

- Follow all directions on the label and in the package.
- Do a patch test on your skin every time before dyeing your hair.
- Keep hair dyes away from your eyes, and do not dye your eyebrows or eyelashes. This can hurt your eyes and may even cause blindness.
- Wear gloves when applying hair dye.
- Do not leave the product on longer than the directions say you should. Keep track of time using a clock or a timer.
- Rinse your scalp well with water after using hair dye.
- Keep hair dyes out of the reach of children.
- Do not scratch or brush your scalp three days before using hair dyes.
- Do not dye or relax your hair if your scalp is irritated, sunburned, or damaged.

- Wait at least 14 days after bleaching, relaxing, or perming your hair before using dye.

- Read the ingredient statement to make certain that ingredients that may have caused a problem for you in the past, such as p-phenylenediamine (PPD) are not present.

If you have a problem, tell your healthcare provider. Then, please report it to FDA.

How To Report A Problem

If you have a reaction to a hair dye—or any other cosmetic—first contact your healthcare provider for any necessary medical help. Then, please tell FDA. The law doesn't require cosmetic companies, including hair dye manufacturers, to share their safety data or consumer complaints with FDA. So, the information you report is very important to help FDA monitor the safety of cosmetics on the market.

You can report a problem with a cosmetic to FDA in either of these ways:

1. Contact MedWatch, FDA's problem reporting program, at 800-332-1088, or file a MedWatch Voluntary report online

2. Contact the consumer complaint coordinator in your area.

Chapter 44

Fragrance Allergy

Many products we use everyday contain fragrances. Some of these products are regulated as cosmetics by U.S. Food and Drug Administration (FDA). Some belong to other product categories and are regulated differently, depending on how the product is intended to be used.

How To Know If A Fragrance Product Is Regulated As A Cosmetic

If a product is intended to be applied to a person's body to make the person more attractive, it's a cosmetic under the law. Here are some examples of fragrance products that are regulated as cosmetics:

- Perfume

- Cologne

- Aftershave

Fragrance ingredients are also commonly used in other products, such as shampoos, shower gels, shaving creams, and body lotions. Even some products labeled "unscented" may contain fragrance ingredients. This is because the manufacturer may add just enough fragrance to mask the unpleasant smell of other ingredients, without giving the product a noticeable scent.

Some fragrance products that are applied to the body are intended for therapeutic uses, such as treating or preventing disease, or affecting the structure or function of the body. Products intended for this type of use are treated as drugs under the law, or sometimes as both

About This Chapter: This chapter includes text excerpted from "Fragrances In Cosmetics," U.S. Food and Drug Administration (FDA), December 29, 2015.

cosmetics and drugs. Here are some examples of labeling statements that will cause a product containing fragrances to be treated as a drug:

- Easing muscle aches
- Soothing headaches
- Helping people sleep
- Treating colic

Many other products that may contain fragrance ingredients, but are not applied to the body, are regulated by the U.S. Consumer Product Safety Commission (CPSC). Here are some examples:

- Laundry detergents
- Fabric softeners
- Dryer sheets
- Room fresheners
- Carpet fresheners

Statements on labels, marketing claims, consumer expectations, and even some ingredients may determine a product's intended use.

"Essential Oils" And "Aromatherapy"

There is no regulatory definition for "essential oils," although people commonly use the term to refer to certain oils extracted from plants. The law treats Ingredients from plants the same as those from any other source.

For example, "essential oils" are commonly used in so-called "aromatherapy" products. If an "aromatherapy" product is intended to treat or prevent disease, or to affect the structure or function of the body, it's a drug.

Similarly, a massage oil intended to lubricate the skin is a cosmetic. But if claims are made that a massage oil relieves aches or relaxes muscles, apart from the action of the massage itself, it's a drug, or possibly both a cosmetic and a drug.

Safety Requirements

Fragrance ingredients in cosmetics must meet the same requirement for safety as other cosmetic ingredients. The law does not require FDA approval before they go on the market, but they must be safe for consumers when they are used according to labeled directions, or as people customarily use them. Companies and individuals who manufacture or market cosmetics have a legal responsibility for ensuring that their products are safe and properly labeled.

Labeling Of Fragrance Ingredients

If a cosmetic is marketed on a retail basis to consumers, such as in stores, on the Internet, or person-to-person, it must have a list of ingredients. In most cases, each ingredient must be listed individually. But under U.S. regulations, fragrance and flavor ingredients can be listed simply as "Fragrance" or "Flavor."

FDA requires the list of ingredients under the Fair Packaging and Labeling Act (FPLA). This law is not allowed to be used to force a company to tell "trade secrets." Fragrance and flavor formulas are complex mixtures of many different natural and synthetic chemical ingredients, and they are the kinds of cosmetic components that are most likely to be "trade secrets."

Fragrance Allergies And Sensitivities

Some individuals may be allergic or sensitive to certain ingredients in cosmetics, food, or other products, even if those ingredients are safe for most people. Some components of fragrance formulas may have a potential to cause allergic reactions or sensitivities for some people.

FDA does not have the same legal authority to require allergen labeling for cosmetics as for food. So, if you are concerned about fragrance sensitivities, you may want to choose products that are fragrance free, and check the ingredient list carefully. If consumers have questions, they may choose to contact the manufacturer directly.

Phthalates As Fragrance Ingredient

Phthalates are a group of chemicals used in hundreds of products. The phthalate commonly used in fragrance products is diethyl phthalate, or DEP. DEP does not pose known risks for human health as it is currently used in cosmetics and fragrances.

Chapter 45

Lanolin Allergy

What Is Lanolin?

Lanolin, a natural product most commonly extracted from the fleece of sheep, is widely used in cosmetic and pharmaceutical products. It is sometimes also referred to as wool fat, wool wax, and wool grease. About 50 percent of lanolin is made up of wool alcohol, a substance containing allergens that can cause skin rashes and itching. A good emulsifier and excellent emollient, lanolin is frequently used in lotions, hair products, and toiletries.

The use of lanolin traces its roots to ancient Greece, where it was first discovered that the water in which sheep's wool was washed contained an oily substance that proved to be a good emollient or moisturizer. The substance was refined through various treatments and became lanolin. Despite improved purification processes, some impurities still remain, some of which include the allergens.

Types Of Lanolin Allergy

Skin reactions to lanolin-based products are usually mild, but in some cases may be more extreme. Most often, a rash will appear after the application of a lanolin product on the skin, generally on the hands, legs, neck, and face, areas on which these products are commonly used. Small red itchy bumps or scaly patches of skin may denote a mild allergic reaction to lanolin, but more serious reactions can result in swelling and blisters.

About This Chapter: "Lanolin Allergy," © 2017 Omnigraphics. Reviewed November 2017.

Symptoms Of Lanolin Allergy

Symptoms of lanolin allergy often occur during the teen years, although they can go undiagnosed for a long time. Common symptoms include red bumpy rashes or scaly patches on the skin. Some people experience nasal congestion and, in extreme cases, lips or other body parts may swell up. Itchy rashes can also form blisters, which can sometimes be quite painful. Constant overall itchiness may also develop. Skin reactions to lanolin products on the body can appear from few hours to few days. The rashes are usually found in a single area, but over time, they may spread to other parts of the body.

Treatment For Lanolin Allergy

Testing can be done by a healthcare professional, or you can try a simple test yourself. Dermatologists typically administer a patch test using 30-percent wool alcohol and then monitor for a lanolin reaction. In a self-test, small amounts of lanolin can be applied over a small patch of skin and observed for five to seven days to see if the skin changes color or a rash develops. However, self-test is recommended only after consultation with a healthcare provider.

Allergies caused by lanolin products can be prevented by testing cosmetic and skin products on a small patch of skin before use. Products that contain wool alcohol should be avoided unless a dermatologist is consulted before the products are used on skin. A dermatologist should also be informed before ointments or creams are prescribed to a person with a lanolin allergy, since many of these products contain lanolin or related substances.

Some common products that may contain lanolin or wool alcohol include face foundations, lip balms, lipsticks, lip liners, makeup removal creams, nail polish removers, mascaras, eyeliner or eye shadow, shaving creams, sunscreen creams, hairsprays, shoe polishes, leather products, dog shampoos, printer ink, hair removal creams, after-shave lotions, body moisturizers, ointments, diaper creams, hemorrhoid creams, nipple creams, and body lotions.

Testing And Prevention Of Lanolin Allergy

Lanolin allergy can cause rashes or breakouts on skin that are annoying and unsightly, as well as more serious symptoms, like painful blisters. The best possible treatment is prevention itself; however, if a person has used a lanolin-based product and an allergic reaction results, then the first step of treatment would be to stop using that product or any substance that contains such ingredients as wool and wool alcohol or its derivatives. The next step would be to consult a professional healthcare provider. Topical steroids and oral antihistamines are most often used for the treatment of lanolin allergies, although if the reaction is extreme, the doctor may recommend a longer course of treatment with oral steroids and possibly antibiotics to treat secondary skin infections.

References

1. Cooley, Andrea. "Skin Reaction To Lanolin," Livestrong.com, July 18, 2012.

2. Cynia. "Lanolin Allergy," Instah.com, September 6, 2014.

3. Jacob, Sharon, M.D. "The Lanolin-Wool Wax Alcohol Update," The Dermatologist, February 18, 2014.

4. Ngan, Vanessa. "Allergy To Wood Alcohols," DermNet New Zealand, 2002.

Chapter 46

Formaldehyde Allergy

What Is Formaldehyde?

At room temperature, formaldehyde is a colorless, flammable gas that has a distinct, pungent smell. Small amounts of formaldehyde are naturally produced by plants, animals, and humans.

It is used in the production of fertilizer, paper, plywood, and urea-formaldehyde resins. It is also used as a preservative in some foods and in many household products, such as antiseptics, medicines, and cosmetics.

Sources Of formaldehyde

Formaldehyde is a common chemical that can be emitted from a number of products in the home. Smoking, pressed wood, and particleboard have all been shown to be sources of formaldehyde. Higher formaldehyde levels are usually found in newer homes or homes with new construction. The levels decrease over time. Formaldehyde levels also increase with increases in temperature and humidity.

(Source: "What You Should Know About Formaldehyde," Agency for Toxic Substances and Disease Registry (ATSDR), Centers for Disease Control and Prevention (CDC).)

About This Chapter: This chapter includes text excerpted from "Toxic Substances Portal—Formaldehyde—ToxFAQs," Agency for Toxic Substances and Disease Registry (ATSDR), Centers for Disease Control and Prevention (CDC), May 12, 2015.

What Happens To Formaldehyde When It Enters The Environment?

- Once formaldehyde is in the air, it is quickly broken down, usually within hours.

- Formaldehyde dissolves easily but does not last a long time in water.

- Formaldehyde evaporates from shallow soils.

- Formaldehyde does not buildup in plants and animals.

How Might I Be Exposed To Formaldehyde?

- The primary way you can be exposed to formaldehyde is by breathing air containing it.

- Releases of formaldehyde into the air occur from industries using or manufacturing formaldehyde, wood products (such as particle-board, plywood, and furniture), automobile exhaust, cigarette smoke, paints and varnishes, and carpets and permanent press fabrics.

- Indoor air contains higher levels of formaldehyde than outdoor air. Levels of formaldehyde measured in indoor air range from 0.02–4 parts per million (ppm). Formaldehyde levels in outdoor air range from 0.0002 to 0.006 ppm in rural and suburban areas and 0.001 to 0.02 ppm in urban areas.

- Breathing contaminated workplace air. The highest potential exposure occurs in the formaldehyde-based resins industry.

Formaldehyde can make you feel sick if you breathe a lot of it. People can have symptoms such as:

- sore throat
- Cough
- scratchy eyes
- Nosebleeds

(Source: "What You Should Know About Formaldehyde," Agency for Toxic Substances and Disease Registry (ATSDR), Centers for Disease Control and Prevention (CDC).)

How Can Formaldehyde Affect My Health?

Nasal and eye irritation, neurological effects, and increased risk of asthma and/or allergy have been observed in humans breathing 0.1 to 0.5 ppm. Eczema and changes in lung function have been observed at 0.6 to 1.9 ppm.

Decreased body weight, gastrointestinal ulcers, liver and kidney damage were observed in animals orally exposed to 50–100 milligrams/kilogram/day (mg/kg/day) formaldehyde.

How Likely Is Formaldehyde To Cause Cancer?

The U.S. Department of Health and Human Services (HHS) determined in 2011 that formaldehyde is a known human carcinogen based on sufficient human and animal inhalation studies.

How Can Formaldehyde Affect Children?

A small number of studies have looked at the health effects of formaldehyde in children. It is very likely that breathing formaldehyde will result in nose and eye irritation. It's not clearly known if the irritation would occur at lower concentrations in children than in adults.

There is some evidence of asthma or asthma-like symptoms for children exposed to formaldehyde in homes.

Animal studies have suggested that formaldehyde will not cause birth defects in humans.

How Can Families Reduce The Risk Of Exposure To Formaldehyde?

Formaldehyde is usually found in the air, and levels are usually higher indoors than outdoors. Opening windows and using fans to bring fresh air indoors are the easiest ways to lower levels in the house. Not smoking and not using unvented heaters indoors can lower the formaldehyde levels.

Formaldehyde is given off from a number of products used in the home. Removing formaldehyde sources in the home can reduce exposure. Providing fresh air, sealing unfinished manufactured wood surfaces, and washing new permanent press clothing before wearing can help lower exposure.

Is There A Medical Test To Show Whether I've Been Exposed To Formaldehyde?

Formaldehyde cannot be reliably measured in blood, urine, or body tissues following exposure. Formaldehyde is produced in the body and would be present as a normal constituent in body tissues and fluids.

Has The Federal Government Made Recommendations To Protect Human Health?

The U.S. Environmental Protection Agency (EPA) has determined that exposure to formaldehyde in drinking water at concentrations of 10 milligrams/liter (mg/L) for 1 day or 5 mg/L for 10 days is not expected to cause any adverse effects in children.

The U.S. EPA has also determined that a lifetime exposure to 1 mg/L of formaldehyde in drinking water is not expected to cause any adverse health effects.

The Occupational Health and Safety Administration (OSHA) has limited workers' exposure to an average of 0.75 ppm for an 8-hour workday, 40-hour workweek.

The U.S. Department of Housing and Urban Development (HUD) has set standards for formaldehyde emissions in manufactured housing of less than 0.2 ppm for plywood and 0.3 ppm for particleboard. The HUD standards are designed to provide an ambient air level of 0.4 ppm or less in manufactured housing.

Part Five
Managing Allergies In Daily Life

Chapter 47

When Breathing Becomes Bothersome

Seasonal Changes Can Cause Breathing Problem

A change in season can brighten your days with vibrant new colors. But blooming flowers and falling leaves can usher in more than beautiful backdrops. Airborne substances that irritate your nose can blow in with the weather. When sneezing, itchy eyes, or a runny nose suddenly appears, allergies may be to blame.

Overreaction Of The Immune System

Allergies are an overreaction of the immune system to substances that generally do not affect other individuals. These substances, or allergens, can cause sneezing, coughing, and itching. Allergic reactions range from merely bothersome to life threatening. Some allergies are seasonal, like hay fever. Allergies have also been associated with chronic conditions like sinusitis and asthma.

(Source: "Allergies," Centers for Disease Control and Prevention (CDC).)

What Causes Allergy?

Allergies arise when the body's immune system overreacts to substances, called allergens, that are normally harmless. When a person with allergies breathes in allergens—such as pollen,

---

About This Chapter: This chapter includes text excerpted from "Seeking Allergy Relief," *NIH News in Health*, National Institutes of Health (NIH), June 2016.

mold, pet dander, or dust mites—the resulting allergic reactions in the nose are called allergic rhinitis, or hay fever.

Allergy is one of the most common long-term health conditions. "Over the past several decades, the prevalence of allergies has been increasing," says Dr. Paivi Salo, an allergy expert at National Institutes of Health (NIH). "Currently, airborne allergies affect approximately 10–30 percent of adults and 40 percent of children."

Avoiding Allergy Triggers

Avoiding your allergy triggers is the best way to control your symptoms. But triggers aren't always easy to identify. Notice when and where your symptoms occur. This can help you figure out the cause.

"Most people with allergies are sensitive to more than one allergen," Salo explains. "Grass, weed, and tree pollens are the most common causes of outdoor allergies." Pollen is often the source if your symptoms are seasonal. Indoor allergens usually trigger symptoms that last all year.

Managing Allergy

If your symptoms become persistent and bothersome, visit your family physician or an allergist. They can test for allergy sensitivities by using a skin or blood test. The test results, along with a medical exam and information about when and where your symptoms occur, will help your doctor determine the cause.

Even when you know your triggers, avoiding allergens can be difficult. When pollen counts are high, stay inside with the windows closed and use the air conditioning. Avoid bringing pollen indoors. "If you go outside, wash your hair and clothing," Salo says. Pets can also bring in pollen, so clean them too.

For indoor allergens, keep humidity levels low in the home to keep dust mites and mold under control. Avoid upholstered furniture and carpets because they harbor allergens. Wash your bedding in hot water, and vacuum the floors once a week.

Allergies run in families. Your children's chances of developing allergies are higher if you have them. While there's no "magic bullet" to prevent allergies, experts recommend breastfeeding early in life. "Breast milk is the least likely to trigger allergic reactions, it's easy to digest, and it strengthens an infant's immune system," Salo says.

Treating Allergies

Sometimes, avoiding allergens isn't possible or isn't enough. Untreated allergies are associated with chronic conditions like sinus infections and asthma. Over-the-counter (OTC) antihistamines, nasal sprays, and decongestants can often ease mild symptoms. Prescription medications and allergy shots are sometimes needed for more severe allergies. Talk with your doctor about treatment options.

Allergy relief can help clear up more than just itchy, watery eyes. It can allow you to breathe easy again and brighten your outlook on seasonal changes.

Anaphylaxis

Anaphylaxis is the most severe allergic reaction. Symptoms include flush; tingling of the palms of the hands, soles of the feet or lips; light-headedness, and chest-tightness. If not treated, these can progress into seizures, cardiac arrhythmia, shock, and respiratory distress. Anaphylaxis can result in death. Food, latex, insect sting, and drug allergies can all result in anaphylaxis.

(Source: "Allergies," Centers for Disease Control and Prevention (CDC).)

Chapter 48

How To Control Seasonal Allergies

Allergic reactions occur when the body wrongly defends itself against something that is not dangerous. A healthy immune system defends against invading bacteria and viruses. During allergic reactions, however, the immune system fights harmless materials, such as pollen or mold, with production of a special class of antibody called immunoglobulin E (IgE).

Treat respiratory allergy with antihistamines, topical nasal steroids, cromolyn sodium, decongestants, or immunotherapy.

Fast Facts

Allergies are reactions of your immune system to one or more things in the environment.

The immune system is your body's defense system. In allergic reactions, however, it is responding to a false alarm.

Pollens and mold spores can cause seasonal allergies.

Allergies from pollens and molds can cause runny and blocked noses, sneezing, nose and eye itching, runny and red eyes rashes, or asthma. Allergies typically make you feel bad.

(Source: "Fast Facts," National Institute of Allergy and Infectious Diseases (NIAID).)

Plant Pollen

Ragweed and other weeds, such as curly dock, lambs quarters, pigweed, plantain, sheep sorrel, and sagebrush are prolific producers of pollen allergens. Ragweed season runs from August

---

About This Chapter: This chapter includes text excerpted from "How To Control Your Seasonal Allergies," MedlinePlus, National Institutes of Health (NIH), April 25, 2013. Reviewed November 2017.

to November, but pollen levels usually peak by mid-September in many areas in the country. Pollen counts are highest in the morning, and on dry, hot, windy days.

Protecting Yourself

- Between 5:00 and 10:00 in the morning, stay indoors. Save outside activities for late afternoon or after a heavy rain, when pollen levels are lower.

- Keep windows in your home and car closed to lower exposure to pollen. Keep cool with air conditioners. Don't use window or attic fans.

- Use a dryer, not a line outside; dry your clothes and avoid collecting pollen on them.

Grass Pollen

Grass pollens are regional as well as seasonal. Their levels also are affected by temperature, time of day, and rain. Only a small percentage of North America's 1,200 grass species cause allergies, including:

- Bermuda grass

- Johnson grass

- Kentucky bluegrass

- Sweet vernal grass

- Timothy grass

- Orchard grass

Protecting Yourself

- Between 5:00 and 10:00 a.m., stay indoors. Save outside activities for late afternoon or after a heavy rain, when pollen levels are lower.

- Keep windows in your home and car closed to lower exposure to pollen. Keep cool with air conditioners. Don't use window or attic fans.

- Use a clothes dryer, not a line outside, to avoid collecting pollen on them.

- Have someone else mow your lawn. If you mow, wear a mask.

Tree Pollen

Trees produce pollen earliest, as soon as January in the south, and as late as May and June in the northeast. They release huge amounts that can be distributed miles away. Fewer than 100 kinds of trees cause allergies. The most common tree allergy is against oak, but others include catalpa, elm, hickory, sycamore, and walnut.

Protecting Yourself

- Follow the same protective strategies related to time of day, closed windows, and clothes dryers noted in "Protecting yourself" under Grass Pollen, above.

- Plant species that do not aggravate allergies, such as crape myrtle, dogwood, fig, fir, palm, pear, plum, redbud, and redwood trees, or the female cultivars of ash, box elder, cotton-wood, maple, palm, poplar, or willow trees.

Seasonal Allergies: Nuisance Or Real Health Threat?

For most people, hay fever is a seasonal problem—something to endure for a few weeks once or twice a year. But for others, such allergies can lead to more serious complications, including sinusitis and asthma.

- Sinusitis is one of the most commonly reported chronic diseases and costs almost $6 billion a year to manage. It is caused by inflammation or infection of the four pairs of cavities behind the nose. Congestion in them can lead to pressure and pain over the eyes, around the nose, or in the cheeks just above the teeth. Chronic sinusitis is associated with persistent inflammation and is often difficult to treat. Extended bouts of hay fever can increase the likelihood of chronic sinusitis. But only half of all people with chronic sinusitis have allergies.

- Asthma is a lung disease that narrows or blocks the airways. This causes wheezing, shortness of breath, coughing, and other breathing difficulties. Asthma attacks can be triggered by viral infections, cold air, exercise, anxiety, allergens, and other factors. Almost 80 percent of people with asthma have allergies, but it's not clearly known to what extent the allergies trigger the breathing problems. However, some people are diagnosed with allergic asthma because the problem is set off primarily by an immune response to one or more specific allergens. Most of the time, the culprit allergens are those found indoors, such as pets, house dust mites, cockroaches, and mold. Increased pollen and mold levels have also been associated with worsening asthma.

Chapter 49

Managing Indoor Air Quality

Biological Contaminants

Biological contaminants include bacteria, viruses, animal dander and cat saliva, house dust, mites, cockroaches, and pollen. There are many sources of these pollutants. By controlling the relative humidity level in a home, the growth of some sources of biologicals can be minimized. A relative humidity of 30–50 percent is generally recommended for homes. Standing water, water damaged materials or wet surfaces also serve as a breeding ground for molds, mildews, bacteria, and insects. House dust mites, the source of one of the most powerful biological allergens, grow in damp, warm environments.

Sources

- pollens, which originate from plants.

- viruses, which are transmitted by people and animals.

- mold.

- bacteria, which are carried by people, animals, and soil and plant debris.

- household pets, which are sources of saliva and animal dander (skin flakes).

- droppings and body parts from cockroaches, rodents and other pests or insects.

- viruses and bacteria.

About This Chapter: This chapter includes text excerpted from "Indoor Air Quality (IAQ)—Biological Pollutants' Impact On Indoor Air Quality," U.S. Environmental Protection Agency (EPA), September 6, 2017.

- the protein in urine from rats and mice is a potent allergen. When it dries, it can become airborne.

- contaminated central air handling systems can become breeding grounds for mold, mildew and other sources of biological contaminants and can then distribute these contaminants through the home.

Many of these biological contaminants are small enough to be inhaled.

Biological contaminants are, or are produced by, living things. Biological contaminants are often found in areas that provide food and moisture or water. For example:

- damp or wet areas such as cooling coils, humidifiers, condensate pans, or unvented bathrooms can be moldy

- draperies, bedding, carpet and other areas where dust collects may accumulate biological contaminants

Health Effects From Biological Contaminants

Some biological contaminants trigger allergic reactions, including:

- hypersensitivity pneumonitis

- allergic rhinitis

- some types of asthma

Infectious illnesses, such as influenza, measles, and chickenpox are transmitted through the air. Molds and mildews release disease causing toxins. Symptoms of health problems caused by biological pollutants include:

- sneezing

- watery eyes

- coughing

- shortness of breath

- dizziness

- lethargy

- fever

- and digestive problems

Allergic reactions occur only after repeated exposure to a specific biological allergen. However, that reaction may occur immediately upon re-exposure or after multiple exposures over time. As a result, people who have noticed only mild allergic reactions, or no reactions at all, may suddenly find themselves very sensitive to particular allergens.

Some diseases, like humidifier fever, are associated with exposure to toxins from microorganisms that can grow in large building ventilation systems. However, these diseases can also be traced to microorganisms that grow in home heating and cooling systems and humidifiers. Children, elderly people, and people with breathing problems, allergies, and lung diseases are particularly susceptible to disease causing biological agents in the indoor air.

Mold, dust mites, pet dander and pest droppings, or body parts can trigger asthma. Biological contaminants, including molds and pollens can cause allergic reactions for a significant portion of the population. Tuberculosis, measles, staphylococcus infections, Legionella and influenza are known to be transmitted by air.

Reducing Exposure To Biological Contaminants

General good housekeeping, and maintenance of heating and air conditioning equipment, are very important. Adequate ventilation and good air distribution also help. The key to mold control is moisture control. If mold is a problem, clean up the mold and get rid of excess water or moisture. Maintaining the relative humidity between 30 percent–60 percent will help control mold, dust mites, and cockroaches. Employ integrated pest management to control insect and animal allergens. Cooling tower treatment procedures exist to reduce levels of Legionella and other organisms.

- **Install and use exhaust fans that are vented to the outdoors in kitchens and bathrooms and vent clothes dryers outdoors.** These actions can eliminate much of the moisture that builds up from everyday activities. There are exhaust fans on the market that produce little noise, an important consideration for some people. Another benefit to using kitchen and bathroom exhaust fans is that they can reduce levels of organic pollutants that vaporize from hot water used in showers and dishwashers.

- **Ventilate the attic and crawl spaces to prevent moisture buildup.** Keeping humidity levels in these areas below 50 percent can prevent water condensation on building materials.

- **If using cool mist or ultrasonic humidifiers, clean appliances according to manufacturer's instructions and refill with fresh water daily.** Because these humidifiers can become breeding grounds for biological contaminants, they have the potential for causing diseases such as hypersensitivity pneumonitis and humidifier fever. Evaporation trays in air conditioners, dehumidifiers, and refrigerators should also be cleaned frequently.

- **Thoroughly clean and dry water damaged carpets and building materials (within 24 hours if possible) or consider removal and replacement.** Water damaged carpets and building materials can harbor mold and bacteria. It is very difficult to completely rid such materials of biological contaminants.

- **Keep the house clean.** House dust mites, pollens, animal dander, and other allergy causing agents can be reduced, although not eliminated, through regular cleaning. People who are allergic to these pollutants should use allergen proof mattress encasements, wash bedding in hot (130°F) water and avoid room furnishings that accumulate dust, especially if they cannot be washed in hot water. Allergic individuals should also leave the house while it is being vacuumed because vacuuming can actually increase airborne levels of mite allergens and other biological contaminants. Using central vacuum systems that are vented to the outdoors or vacuums with high efficiency filters may also be of help.

- **Take steps to minimize biological pollutants in basements.** Clean and disinfect the basement floor drain regularly. Do not finish a basement below ground level unless all water leaks are patched and outdoor ventilation and adequate heat to prevent condensation are provided. Operate a dehumidifier in the basement if needed to keep relative humidity levels between 30–50 percent.

Improving Your Indoor Air

Take steps to help improve your air quality and reduce your Indoor air quality (IAQ) related health risks at little or no cost by:

- **Controlling the sources of pollution:** Usually the most effective way to improve indoor air is to eliminate individual sources or reduce their emissions.

- **Ventilating:** Increasing the amount of fresh air brought indoors helps reduce pollutants inside. When weather permits, open windows and doors, or run an air conditioner with the vent control open. Bathroom and kitchen fans that exhaust to the outdoors also increase ventilation and help remove pollutants.

Opening windows and doors, operating window or attic fans, when the weather permits, or running a window air conditioner with the vent control open increases the outdoor ventilation rate. Local bathroom or kitchen fans that exhaust outdoors remove contaminants directly from the room where the fan is located and also increase the outdoor air ventilation rate.

(Source: "Improving Indoor Air Quality," U.S. Environmental Protection Agency (EPA).)

- Always ventilate and follow manufacturers' instructions when you use products or appliances that may release pollutants into the indoor air.

- **Changing filters regularly:** Central heaters and air conditioners have filters to trap dust and other pollutants in the air. Make sure to change or clean the filters regularly, following the instructions on the package.

- **Adjusting humidity:** The humidity inside can affect the concentrations of some indoor air pollutants. For example, high humidity keeps the air moist and increases the likelihood of mold.

Keep indoor humidity between 30 and 50 percent. Use a moisture or humidity gauge, available at most hardware stores, to see if the humidity in your home is at a good level. To increase humidity, use a vaporizer or humidifier. To decrease humidity, open the windows if it is not humid outdoors. If it is warm, turn on the air conditioner or adjust the humidity setting on the humidifier.

Take Action To Improve Air Quality In Every Room

Important tips that will help control indoor pollutants:

- Test for radon and fix if there is a problem.

- Reduce asthma triggers such as mold and dust mites.

- Do not let people smoke indoors.

- Keep all areas clean and dry. Clean up any mold and get rid of excess water or moisture.

- Always ventilate when using products that can release pollutants into the air; if products must be stored following use, make sure to close tightly.

- Inspect fuel burning appliances regularly for leaks, and make repairs when necessary.

- Consider installing a carbon monoxide alarm.

Chapter 50

Asthma Management At School

Asthma is a leading chronic illness among children and adolescents in the United States. It is also one of the leading causes of school absenteeism. On average, in a classroom of 30 children, about 3 are likely to have asthma. Low income populations, minorities, and children living in inner cities experience more emergency department visits, hospitalizations, and deaths due to asthma than the general population.

When children and adolescents are exposed to things in the environment—such as dust mites, and tobacco smoke—an asthma episode can occur. These are called asthma triggers. Asthma symptoms can be controlled by avoiding triggers and taking medications prescribed by a healthcare provider, if needed. Asthma is common but treatable: using treatment based on current scientific knowledge reduces illness and future episodes.

Asthma And School Attendance

Many schools have shown a high incidence of students missing valuable school days due to asthma and allergies. In many of the same schools that report a high incidence of absenteeism, the cockroach infestations in cafeterias, storage closets, and teacher break rooms are also found.

Is there a relationship between cockroach exposure, allergies and asthma?

Most people with asthma have allergic responses in their bronchial tubes when they breathe in particles of the right size and shape and composed of materials recognized by their immune

About This Chapter: Text in this chapter begins with excerpts from "Healthy Schools—Asthma In Schools," Centers for Disease Control and Prevention (CDC), May 9, 2017; Text under the heading "Controlling Common Asthma Triggers Found In Schools" is excerpted from "Managing Asthma In The School Environment," U.S. Environmental Protection Agency (EPA), March 15, 2017.

system. Exposure to things like mold, cat dander, ragweed, pollen, and rodent and cockroach droppings can elicit an allergic reaction.

The proteins in cockroach feces and their decomposing bodies are of just the right size to be lifted into the air, inhaled and recognized by the immune system as a signal to make an allergic reaction in some people. This is asthma. Airborne cockroach allergens will stick to particles, like dust, that quickly settle onto dust-trapping fabrics found on upholstered furniture, carpets and curtains. Activities like vacuuming, or even walking may stir up these allergens.

An asthma attack can happen when a student is exposed to "asthma triggers." One child's triggers can be very different from those of another child or an adult with asthma.

(Source: "Children's Health: A Link Between Allergies, Asthma And School Attendance," U.S. Environmental Protection Agency (EPA).)

Managing Asthma In Schools

Asthma friendly schools are those that make the effort to create safe and supportive learning environments for students with asthma. They have policies and procedures that allow students to successfully manage their asthma. Research and case studies that looked at ways to best manage asthma in schools found that successful school based asthma programs.

- Establish strong links with asthma care clinicians to ensure appropriate and ongoing medical care

- Target students who are the most affected by asthma at school to identify and intervene with those in greatest need

- Get administrative buy in and build a team of enthusiastic people, including a full time school nurse, to support the program

- Use a coordinated, multi component and collaborative approach that includes school nursing services, asthma education for students and professional development for school staff

- Provide appropriate school health services for students with asthma, ensuring that students take their medicines and learn to use them when appropriate

- Provide asthma education for students with asthma and awareness programs for students, school staff, parents, and families

- Provide a safe and healthy school environment to reduce asthma triggers

- Offer safe and enjoyable physical education and activities for students with asthma

- Support evaluation of school-based programs and use adequate and appropriate outcome measures

Controlling Common Asthma Triggers Found In Schools

Table 50.1. Managing Asthma In The School Environment

Asthma Triggers Found In Schools	Asthma Management Tips For Schools
Environmental Tobacco Smoke: Environmental tobacco smoke is a mixture of smoke from the burning end of a cigarette, pipe, or cigar and the smoke exhaled by the smoker.	**Eliminate Exposure to Environmental Tobacco Smoke.** Enforce no-smoking policies in schools.
Pests: Cockroach body parts, secretions, and droppings, as well as the urine, droppings, and saliva of other pests (such as rodents) are often found in areas where food and water are present.	**Control Pest Problems.** Use Integrated Pest Management (IPM) to prevent cockroach and other pest problems (e.g., store food in tightly sealed containers and place dumpsters away from the building).
Mold: Mold can grow indoors when mold spores land on wet or damp surfaces. In schools, mold is most commonly found in bathrooms, kitchens, basements, around roof seams and plumbing, and in portable classrooms and trailers. Mold can grow anywhere that moisture is present.	**Clean Up Mold and Moisture.** Fix leaks and moisture problems and thoroughly dry wet areas within 24–48 hours to prevent mold growth. Clean hard, moldy surfaces with water and detergent, then dry thoroughly.
Dust mites: Dust mites are too small to be seen but can be found in almost every home, school, and building. Dust mites can be found in school carpeting, upholstered furniture, stuffed animals or toys, and pillows.	**Reduce Dust Mite Exposure.** Make sure schools are dusted and vacuumed thoroughly and regularly, and keep classrooms free of clutter. If stuffed toys are present, ensure they are washable and wash them regularly in hot water.
Animal dander: Pets' skin flakes, urine, and saliva are often found in classrooms and science labs. Any warm-blooded animal, including cats and dogs, may trigger asthma.	**Control Animal Allergens.** Remove classroom animals from the school, if possible. If not, locate animals away from sensitive students and ventilation systems.

Chapter 51

Using Cosmetics Safely

People use cosmetics to keep clean and enhance their beauty. These products range from lipstick and nail polish to deodorant, perfume, hairspray, shampoo, shower gel, tattoos, hair adhesives, hair removal products, hair dyes, most soaps, some tooth whiteners, and some cleansing wipes. It's important to use cosmetics products safely.

The U.S. Food and Drug Administration (FDA) reminds you to get the facts before using cosmetics products.

General Tips

Follow these safety guidelines when using cosmetics products of any type:

- **Read the label.** Follow all directions and heed all warnings.
- **Wash your hands** before you use the product.
- **Do not share makeup.**
- Keep the containers **clean and tightly** closed when not in use, and protect them from temperature extremes.
- Throw away cosmetics if there are **changes in color or smell**.
- Use aerosols or sprays cans in **well ventilated areas**. Do not use them while you are smoking or near an open flame. It could start a fire.

About This Chapter: This chapter includes text excerpted from "Cosmetics—Using Cosmetics Safely," U.S. Food and Drug Administration (FDA), August 25, 2015.

Eye Makeup Tips

There are special safety guidelines for using cosmetics in the eye area. Be sure to keep these practices in mind:

- Do not use cosmetics near your eyes unless they are meant for your eyes. For example, do not use lip liner on your eyes.

- Do not add saliva or water to mascara. You could add germs.

- Throw away your eye makeup if you get an eye infection. The makeup could have become contaminated.

- Do not dye or tint your eyelashes. FDA has not approved any products for permanent dyeing or tinting of your eyelashes or eyebrows.

> Most eye cosmetics are safe when used properly. However, it's important to be careful about the risk of infection, injury from the applicator, and use of unapproved color additives.
>
> *(Source: "Eye Cosmetic Safety," U.S. Food and Drug Administration (FDA).)*

Understanding Cosmetic Labels

Being familiar with the product you are using is important. Be sure to read the entire label, including the list of ingredients, warnings, and tips on how to use the product safely. Also, be aware of the following terms that you may see on the label:

- **Hypoallergenic:** Do not assume that the product will not cause allergic reactions. FDA does not define "hypoallergenic."

- **Organic or Natural:** The source of the ingredients does not determine how safe it is. Do not assume that these products are safer than products made with ingredients from other sources. The U.S. Department of Agriculture (USDA) defines what it means for cosmetics to be labeled "organic." However, there is no formal USDA or FDA definition for "natural."

- **Expiration Dates:** The law does not require cosmetics to have an expiration date. However, a cosmetic product may go bad if you store it the wrong way—for example, in a place that is too warm or too moist. Marking the container with the date you open a cosmetic may help you keep track of the age of your cosmetics.

Report Problems To FDA

The law does *not* require cosmetics to be approved by FDA before they are sold in stores. However, FDA *does* monitor consumer reports of adverse events with cosmetic products.

Please notify FDA if you experience a rash, redness, burn, or another unexpected reaction after using a cosmetic product. Also, please contact FDA if you notice a problem with the cosmetic product itself, such as a bad smell, color change, or foreign material in the product.

Follow these steps:

1. Stop using the product.

2. Call your healthcare provider to find out how to take care of the problem.

3. Report problems to FDA in either of these ways:

   • Contact **MedWatch**, FDA's Safety Information and Adverse Event Reporting Program:

     1. By Phone: 800-FDA-1088

     2. Online: File a voluntary report

   • Contact the Consumer Complaint Coordinator in your area.

Chapter 52

Use Caution With Face Painting And Tattoos

Face paints can be fun on Halloween and other special occasions. Here are tips to help keep your fun from leaving you with a rash, swollen eyelids, or other reaction.

Painting Your Face: Special Effects Without After Effects

Decorating your face with face paint or other makeup lets you see better than you can if you're wearing a mask. A mask can make it hard to see where you're going and watch out for cars. But make sure your painted on designs don't cause problems of their own.

- Follow all directions carefully.

- Don't decorate your face with things that aren't intended for your skin.

- If your face paint has a very bad smell, this could be a sign that it is contaminated. Throw it away and use another one.

- Like soap, some things are OK on your skin, but not in your eyes. Some face paint or other makeup may say on the label that it is not for use near the eyes. Believe this, even if the label has a picture of people wearing it near their eyes. Be careful to keep makeup from getting into your eyes.

About This Chapter: Text beginning with the heading "Painting Your Face: Special Effects Without After Effects" is excerpted from "Cosmetics—Novelty Makeup," U.S. Food and Drug Administration (FDA), February 29, 2016; Text beginning with the heading "Should I Be Concerned About Unsafe Practices, Or The Tattoo Ink Itself?" is excerpted from "For Consumers—Think Before You Ink: Are Tattoos Safe?" U.S. Food and Drug Administration (FDA), May 2, 2017.

- Even products intended for use near your eyes can sometimes irritate your skin if you use too much.

- If you're decorating your skin with something you've never used before, you might try a dab of it on your arm for a couple of days to check for an allergic reaction **BEFORE** you put it on your face. This is an especially smart thing to do if you tend to have allergies.

Color Additives: The "U.S. Food And Drug Administration (FDA) OK" (Or, A Little Detective Work Won't Hurt)

A big part of Halloween makeup is color. But this is your skin we're talking about. Think about what you're putting on it. You might not want to put the same coloring on your skin that a car company uses in its paint.

Luckily, you don't have to. The law says that color additives have to be approved by the FDA for use in cosmetics, including color additives in face paints and other cosmetics that may be used around Halloween time. It also includes theatrical makeup.

Plus, FDA has to decide how they may be used, based on safety information. A color that's OK on your tough fingernails or your hair may not be OK on your skin. Colors that are OK for most of your skin may not be OK near your eyes.

How do you know which ones are OK to use, and where? Do some detective work and check two places:

1. The list of ingredients on the label. Look for the names of the colors.

2. Check the Summary of Color Additives on FDA's website. There's a section especially on colors for cosmetics. If there's a color in your makeup that isn't on this list, the company that made it is not obeying the law. Don't use it. Even if it's on the list, check to see if it has FDA's OK for use near the eyes. If it doesn't, keep it away from your eyes.

For That Ghoulish Glow

There are two kinds of "glow" effects you might get from Halloween type makeup. Ready for some ten-dollar words? There are "fluorescent" and "luminescent" colors.

Here's the difference:

- **Fluorescent colors:** These are the make you blink colors sometimes called "neon" or "day glow." There are eight fluorescent colors approved for cosmetics, and like other colors, there are limits on how they may be used. None of them are allowed for use near the eyes.

- **Luminescent colors:** These colors glow in the dark. In August 2000, FDA approved luminescent zinc sulfide for limited cosmetic use. It's the only luminescent color approved for cosmetic use, and it's not for every day and not for near your eyes. You can recognize it by its whitish yellowish greenish glow.

When The Party's Over

Don't go to bed with your makeup on. Wearing it too long might irritate your skin, and bits of makeup can flake off or smear and get into your eyes, not to mention mess up your pillow and annoy your parents.

How you take the stuff off is as important as how you put it on. Remove it the way the label says. If it says to remove it with cold cream, use cold cream. If it says to remove it with soap and water, use soap and water. If it says to remove it with eye makeup remover, use eye makeup remover. You get the picture. The same goes for removing glue, like the stuff that holds on fake beards.

And remember, the skin around your eyes is delicate. Remove makeup gently.

But Just In Case

What if you followed all these steps and still had a bad reaction? If you have a reaction that seems to be caused by face paints, your parents may want to call a doctor, and they can call FDA, too. To report a bad reaction to face paint, novelty makeup, or any other cosmetic product.

Tattoos are more popular than ever. According to a 2015 Harris Poll, about 3 in 10 (or 29%) people surveyed have at least one tattoo. The FDA is also seeing reports of people developing infections from contaminated tattoo inks, as well as adverse reactions to the inks themselves.

Over the years, the FDA has received hundreds of adverse event reports involving tattoos: 363 from 2004–2016.

Should I Be Concerned About Unsafe Practices, Or The Tattoo Ink Itself?

Both. While you can get serious infections from unhygienic practices and equipment that isn't sterile, infections can also result from ink that was contaminated with bacteria or mold. Using nonsterile water to dilute the pigments (ingredients that add color) is a common culprit, although not the only one.

There's no sure fire way to tell if the ink is safe. An ink can be contaminated even if the container is sealed or the label says the product is sterile.

What Is In Tattoo Ink?

Published research has reported that some inks contain pigments used in printer toner or in car paint. FDA has not approved any pigments for injection into the skin for cosmetic purposes.

FDA reviews reports of adverse reactions or infections from consumers and healthcare providers.

What Kinds Of Reactions May Happen After Getting A Tattoo?

You might notice a rash—redness or bumps—in the area of your tattoo, and you could develop a fever.

More aggressive infections may cause high fever, shaking, chills, and sweats. Treating such infections might require a variety of antibiotics—possibly for months—or even hospitalization and/or surgery. A rash may also mean you're having an allergic reaction. And because the inks are permanent, the reaction may persist.

Can Scar Tissue Buildup After Getting A Tattoo?

Scar tissue may form when you get a tattoo, or you could develop "granulomas," small knots or bumps that may form around material that the body perceives as foreign. If you tend to get keloids—scars that grow beyond normal boundaries—you may develop the same kind of reaction to the tattoo.

What Do I Need To Know About Magnetic Resonance Imaging (MRI) If I Get A Tattoo?

Some people may have swelling or burning in the tattoo when they have magnetic resonance imaging (MRI), although this happens rarely and does not last long. Let your healthcare professional know that you have a tattoo before an MRI is ordered.

What About Do It Yourself Tattoo Inks And Kits?

Inks and kits sold as "do it yourself" to consumers have been associated with infections and allergic reactions. FDA is also concerned that consumers may not know how to control and avoid all sources of contamination.

Could Other Problems Occur Later On?

Although research is ongoing at FDA and elsewhere, there are still a lot of questions about the long-term effects of the pigments, other ingredients, and possible contaminants in tattoo inks. FDA has received reports of bad reactions to tattoo inks right after tattooing and even years later. You also might become allergic to other products, such as hair dyes, if your tattoo contains p-phenylenediamene (PPD).

Then there's tattoo removal. The short or long-term consequences of how pigments break down after laser treatment is not known. However, some tattoo removal procedures may leave permanent scarring.

If I Get A Tattoo And Develop An Infection Or Other Reaction, What Should I Do?

First, contact your healthcare professional.

Second, notify the tattoo artist so he or she can identify the ink and avoid using it again. Ask for the brand, color, and any lot or batch number of the ink or diluent to help determine the source of the problem and how to treat it.

Third, whether you're a consumer, tattoo artist, or healthcare professional, tell FDA. Provide as much detail as possible about the ink and your reaction and outcome.

Removing Tattoos May Be Harder Than You Think

So think before you ink. Consider the risks.

Remember, too, that removing a tattoo is a painstaking process, and complete removal without scarring may be impossible.

If you do decide to get a tattoo, make sure the tattoo parlor and artist comply with state and local laws.

Chapter 53

Nail Care Product Safety

Manicures and pedicures can be pretty. The cosmetic products used, such as nail polishes and nail polish removers, also must be safe—and are regulated by the U.S. Food and Drug Administration (FDA).

The FDA also regulates devices used to dry (or "cure") artificial nails or gel nail polish as electronic products because they emit radiation. You can do your part to stay safe (and look polished, too) by following all labeled directions and paying attention to any warning statements listed on these products.

Cosmetic Nail Care Products: Ingredients And Warnings

Cosmetic ingredients (except most color additives) and products, including nail products, do not need FDA approval before they go on the market. But these products are required to be safe when used as intended. (Note that nail products intended to treat medical problems are classified as drugs and do require FDA approval.)

Cosmetic nail care products also must include any instructions or warnings needed to use them safely. For example:

- Some nail products can catch fire easily so you should not expose them to flames (such as from a lit cigarette) or heat sources (such as a curling iron).

About This Chapter: Text in this chapter begins with excerpts from "How To Safely Use Nail Care Products," U.S. Food and Drug Administration (FDA), September 18, 2017; Text beginning with the heading "How Nail Products Are Regulated" is excerpted from "Cosmetics—Nail Care Products," U.S. Food and Drug Administration (FDA), October 26, 2016.

- Some can injure your eyes, so you should avoid this exposure.

- Some should only be used in areas with good air circulation (ventilation).

- Some ingredients can be harmful if swallowed, so these products should never be consumed by any person or pet.

Also know that retail cosmetics such as those sold in stores or online must list ingredients in the order of decreasing amounts. If you're concerned about certain ingredients, you can check the label and avoid using products with those ingredients.

For example, some nail hardeners and nail polishes may contain formaldehyde, which can cause skin irritation or an allergic reaction. And acrylics, used in some artificial nails and sometimes in nail polishes, can cause allergic reactions.

The bottom line? Read the labels of cosmetic products and follow all instructions. And if you go to a salon for a manicure or pedicure, make sure the space has good ventilation.

Note: Nail salon practices are regulated by the states, and not the FDA. If you're a nail salon owner or employee, you can find information on maintaining safe salons on the webpage of the U.S. Department of Labor's (DOL) Occupational and Health Safety Administration (OSHA).

If you have questions about whether certain nail products are right for you, talk to your healthcare provider.

About Nail Drying And Curing Lamps—And UV Exposure

Ultraviolet (UV) nail curing lamps are table-top size units used to dry or "cure" acrylic or gel nails and gel nail polish. These devices are used in salons and sold online. They feature lamps or LEDs that emit UV (ultraviolet) radiation. (Nail curing lamps are different than sunlamps, which are sometimes called "tanning beds."

Exposure to UV radiation can cause damage to your skin, especially if you're exposed over time. For example, it can lead to premature wrinkles, age spots, and even skin cancer.

But the FDA views nail curing lamps as low risk when used as directed by the label. For example, a study indicated that—even for the worst-case lamp that was evaluated—36 minutes of daily exposure to this lamp was below the occupational exposure limits for UV radiation. (Note that these limits only apply to normal, healthy people and not to people who may have a condition that makes them extra sensitive to UV radiation.)

You may particularly want to avoid these lamps if you're using certain medications or supplements that make you more sensitive to UV rays. These medications include some antibiotics, oral contraceptives, and estrogens—and supplements can include St. John's Wort.

Also remove cosmetics, fragrances, and skin care products (except sunscreen!) before using these lamps, as some of these products can make you more sensitive to UV rays.

If you have questions about using nail drying or curing lamps, consult a healthcare professional.

And if you do choose to use these devices, you can reduce UV exposure by:

• Wearing UV-absorbing gloves that expose only your nails.

• Wearing a broad-spectrum sunscreen with a sun protection factor (SPF) of 15 or higher. (Since nail treatments can include exposure to water, follow the sunscreen's labeled directions for use in these situations.)

Finally, nail curing lamps usually come with instructions for exposure time. The shorter your exposure, the less risky the exposure, in general. So always follow labeled directions when available. In general, you should not use these devices for more than 10 minutes per hand, per session.

How Nail Products Are Regulated

Nail products for both home and salon use are regulated by the FDA. Under the Federal Food, Drug, and Cosmetic Act (FD&C Act), these products are generally regulated as cosmetics [FD&C Act, section 201(i)].

Nail products intended to treat medical problems, such as nail fungus, are drugs.

By law, nail products sold in the United States must be safe for consumers when used according to directions on the label, or in the usual or customary way. Many nail products contain potentially harmful ingredients, but are allowed on the market because they are safe when used as directed. For example, some nail ingredients are harmful when swallowed, but not when used on the nails, because the nail is a barrier, which prevents absorption.

The labels of all cosmetics, whether marketed to consumers or salons, must include a warning statement whenever necessary or appropriate to prevent a health hazard that may occur with use of the product (21 The Code of Federal Regulations (CFR) 740.1).

Cosmetics sold on a retail basis to consumers, such in stores or online, must also bear a list of ingredients, with the names of the ingredients listed in descending order of predominance.

The requirement for an ingredient declaration does not apply, for example, to products used only at salons and to free samples. However, the products must have a list of ingredients if they are also sold at retail, even if they are labeled "For professional use only."

Under the law, cosmetic products and ingredients, including nail products, do not need FDA approval before they go on the market, with the exception of most color additives. However, FDA may take action against cosmetics that do not comply with the law, or against firms or individuals who violate the enforced laws.

While FDA regulates the nail products intended for use at home and in salons, state and local authorities regulate the operation of nail salons and the licensing of manicurists and nail technicians. Also, the OSHA has addressed the safety of employees in nail salons.

Chapter 54

Skin Care Concerns For People With Eczema

Atopic dermatitis is a skin disease. When a person has this disease the skin becomes extremely itchy. Scratching leads to redness, swelling, cracking, "weeping" clear fluid, crusting, and scaling. Often, the skin gets worse (flares), and then it improves or clears up (remissions).

Atopic dermatitis is the most common kind of eczema, a term that describes many kinds of skin problems.

> ## Who Gets It?
>
> Atopic dermatitis is most common in babies and children. But it can happen to anyone. People who live in cities and dry climates may be more likely to get this disease.
>
> You can't "catch" the disease or give it to other people.

What Are The Symptoms?

The most common symptoms of atopic dermatitis are:

- Dry and itchy skin.

- Rashes on the face, inside the elbows, behind the knees, and on the hands and feet.

About This Chapter: Text in this chapter begins with excerpts from "Atopic Dermatitis," National Institute of Arthritis and Musculoskeletal and Skin Diseases (NIAMS), July 31, 2016; Text beginning with the heading "Skin Care At Home" is excerpted from "Eczema—Eczema (Atopic Dermatitis) Treatment," National Institute of Allergy and Infectious Diseases (NIAID), May 24, 2017.

Scratching the skin can cause:

- Redness.

- Swelling.

- Cracking.

- "Weeping" clear fluid.

- Crusting.

- Thick skin.

- Scaling.

What Causes It?

No one knows what causes atopic dermatitis. It is probably passed down from your parents (genetics). Your environment can also trigger symptoms. Stress can make the condition worse, but it does not cause the disease.

Is There A Test?

Currently, there is no single test to diagnose atopic dermatitis, but your doctor may:

- Ask you about your medical history, including:

    - Your family history of allergies.

    - Whether you also have diseases such as hay fever or asthma.

    - Exposure to irritants, such as:

    - Wool or synthetic fibers.

    - Soaps and detergents.

    - Some perfumes and cosmetics.

    - Substances such as chlorine, mineral oil, or solvents.

    - Dust or sand.

    - Cigarette smoke.

    - Sleep problems.

    - Foods that seem to be related to skin flares.

- Previous treatments for skin-related symptoms.

- Use of steroids or other medications.

- Identify factors that may trigger flares of atopic dermatitis by pricking the skin with a needle that contains something that you might be allergic to (in small amounts).

Your doctor may need to see you several times to diagnose you. In some cases, your family doctor or pediatrician may refer you to a dermatologist (doctor specializing in skin disorders) or allergist (allergy specialist) for further evaluation.

How To Control Atopic Dermatitis?

Besides medications, there are a number of things you can do to help control your atopic dermatitis.

- Skin care: Sticking with a daily skin care routine can prevent flares. Skin care should include:

  - Lukewarm baths to cleanse and moisturize the skin without drying it out.

  - Using mild bar soap or nonsoap cleanser.

  - Air-drying the skin after bathing, or gently patting it dry.

  - A moisturizer to seal in the water after bathing. Use creams and ointments and avoid lotions with high water or alcohol content.

  - Protecting the skin from rough clothing, such as wool or man-made fibers.

- Stay away from things you are allergic to, such as:

  - Dust mites:

  - Put mattresses and pillows inside special dust-proof covers.

  - Wash sheets, blankets, and bed covers often using hot water.

  - Remove carpets.

  - Molds.

  - Pollen.

  - Cat or dog dander.

  - Some perfumes and makeups.

- Certain foods such as eggs, peanuts, milk, fish, soy products, or wheat. You should change your diet to avoid any foods you are allergic to.

- Stress management and relaxation techniques to decrease numbers of flares. Talking to family, friends, health professionals, and support groups can help.

- Prevent scratching or rubbing, which irritates the skin, increases swelling, and actually increases itchiness. Keep your child's fingernails short to help reduce scratching.

Atopic dermatitis and vaccination against smallpox. People with atopic dermatitis should not get the smallpox vaccine. It may cause serious problems in people with atopic dermatitis.

How Is It Treated?

The goals in treating atopic dermatitis are to heal the skin and prevent flares. You should watch for changes in the skin to find out what treatments help the most.

Treatments can include:

- Medications:

    - Skin creams or ointments that control swelling and lower allergic reactions.

    - Corticosteroids.

    - Antibiotics to treat infections caused by bacteria.

    - Antihistamines that make people sleepy to help stop nighttime scratching.

    - Drugs that suppress the immune system.

- Light therapy.

- Skin care that helps heal the skin and keep it healthy.

- Avoiding things that cause an allergic reaction.

Who Treats

Atopic dermatitis may be treated by:

- Family doctors or pediatricians, who can help diagnosis the disease or refer you to specialists.

- Dermatologists, who specialize in skin disorders.

- Allergists, who specialize in allergies.

Skin Care At Home

You and your doctor should discuss the best treatment plan and medications for your atopic dermatitis. But taking care of your skin at home may reduce the need for prescription medications. Some recommendations include:

- Avoid scratching the rash or skin.

- Relieve the itch by using a moisturizer or topical steroids. Take antihistamines to reduce severe itching.

- Keep your fingernails cut short. Consider light gloves if nighttime scratching is a problem.

- Lubricate or moisturize the skin two to three times a day using ointments such as petroleum jelly. Moisturizers should be free of alcohol, scents, dyes, fragrances, and other skin irritating chemicals. A humidifier in the home also can help.

- Avoid anything that worsens symptoms, including:

- Irritants such as wool and lanolin (an oily substance derived from sheep wool used in some moisturizers and cosmetics)

- Strong soaps or detergents

- Sudden changes in body temperature and stress, which may cause sweating

- When washing or bathing

- Keep water contact as brief as possible and use gentle body washes and cleansers instead of regular soaps. Lukewarm baths are better than long, hot baths.

- Do not scrub or dry the skin too hard or for too long.

- After bathing, apply lubricating ointments to damp skin. This will help trap moisture in the skin.

Wet Wrap Therapy

Researchers at National Institute of Allergy and Infectious Diseases (NIAID) and other institutions are studying an innovative treatment for severe eczema called wet wrap therapy. It includes three lukewarm baths a day, each followed by an application of topical medicines and moisturizer that is sealed in by a wrap of wet gauze.

Chapter 55

Have Food Allergies? Read The Label

Food allergy is an abnormal response to a food triggered by your body's immune system.

The allergic reaction may be mild. In rare cases it can cause a severe reaction called anaphylaxis. Symptoms of food allergy include:

- Itching or swelling in your mouth
- Vomiting, diarrhea, or abdominal cramps and pain
- Hives or eczema
- Tightening of the throat and trouble breathing
- Drop in blood pressure

Your healthcare provider may use a detailed history, elimination diet, and skin and blood tests to diagnose a food allergy.

(Source: "Food Allergy," MedlinePlus, National Institutes of Health (NIH).)

Since 2006, it has been much easier for people allergic to certain foods to avoid packaged products that contain them, says Rhonda Kane, a registered dietitian and consumer safety officer at the U.S. Food and Drug Administration (FDA).

This is because a federal law requires that the labels of most packaged foods marketed in the United States disclose—in simple to understand terms—when they are made with a "major food allergen."

About This Chapter: Text in this chapter begins with excerpts from "For Consumers—Have Food Allergies? Read the Label," U.S. Food and Drug Administration (FDA), September 27, 2017; Text beginning with the heading "FDA Steps In" is excerpted from "For Consumers—FDA: Foods Must Contain What Label Says," U.S. Food and Drug Administration (FDA), August 18, 2017.

As someone who cares about what your family eats, you make it a practice when shopping to read the labels on food packages. And you have the right to expect that the information on the label, including the ingredient list, is accurate.

The good news is that the U.S. Food and Drug Administration (FDA) has your back.

The Federal Food, Drug, and Cosmetic Act (FD&C Act)—which provides authority for FDA's consumer protection work—requires that labels on packaged food products in interstate commerce not be false or misleading in any way. To that end, as resources permit, FDA monitors food products to ensure that the labels are truthful and not misleading, explains Michael W. Roosevelt, acting director of compliance at FDA's Center for Food Safety and Applied Nutrition (CFSAN). If a product is not labeled as required by law, the agency takes appropriate action.

Eight foods, and ingredients containing their proteins, are defined as major food allergens. These foods account for 90 percent of all food allergies:

- milk

- egg

- fish, such as bass, flounder, or cod

- crustacean shellfish, such as crab, lobster, or shrimp

- tree nuts, such as almonds, pecans, or walnuts

- wheat

- peanuts

- soybeans

The law allows manufacturers a choice in how they identify the specific "food source names," such as "milk," "cod," "shrimp," or "walnuts," of the major food allergens on the label. They must be declared either in:

- the ingredient list, such as "casein (milk)" or "nonfat dry milk," or

- a separate "Contains" statement, such as "Contains milk," placed immediately after or next to the ingredient list.

"So first look for the 'Contains' statement and if your allergen is listed, put the product back on the shelf," says Kane. "If there is no 'Contains' statement, it's very important to read the entire ingredient list to see if your allergen is present. If you see its name even once, it's back to the shelf for that food too."

There are many different ingredients that contain the same major food allergen, but sometimes the ingredients' names do not indicate their specific food sources. For example, casein, sodium caseinate, and whey are all milk proteins. Although the same allergen can be present in multiple ingredients, its "food source name" (for example, milk) must appear in the ingredient list just once to comply with labeling requirements.

"Contains" And "May Contain" Have Different Meanings

If a "Contains" statement appears on a food label, it must include the food source names of all major food allergens used as ingredients. For example, if "whey," "egg yolks," and a "natural flavor" that contained peanut proteins are listed as ingredients, the "Contains" statement must identify the words "milk," "egg," and "peanuts."

Some manufacturers voluntarily include a "may contain" statement on their labels when there is a chance that a food allergen could be present. A manufacturer might use the same equipment to make different products. Even after cleaning this equipment, a small amount of an allergen (such as peanuts) that was used to make one product (such as cookies) may become part of another product (such as crackers). In this case, the cracker label might state "may contain peanuts."

Be aware that the "may contain" statement is voluntary, says Kane. "You still need to read the ingredient list to see if the product contains your allergen."

When In Doubt, Leave It Out

Manufacturers can change their products' ingredients at any time, so Kane says it's a good idea to check the ingredient list every time you buy the product—even if you have eaten it before and didn't have an allergic reaction.

"If you're unsure about whether a food contains any ingredient to which you are sensitive, don't buy the product, or check with the manufacturer first to ask what it contains," says Kane. "We all want convenience, but it's not worth playing Russian roulette with your life or that of someone under your care."

FDA Steps In

For example, when FDA received complaints from U.S. firms and attorneys alleging that imports of pomegranate juice concentrates were not, as labeled, 100 percent pomegranate, the agency took a closer look.

After conducting its own analyses, FDA found that some of the samples contained undeclared ingredients, including artificial colors, sweeteners and less expensive fruit juices, such as black currant, apple, pear or cherry juices, in place of pomegranate juice.

FDA issued an import alert for pomegranate juice exported by certain companies in Iran and Turkey, based on findings that the samples FDA analyzed were "not as they were represented to be on the labels and therefore adulterated and misbranded." An import alert allows FDA to detain, without physical examination, imported products that appear to violate the Federal Food, Drug, and Cosmetic Act (FFDCA). When a shipment is detained, the importer has a window of opportunity to introduce evidence to overcome the appearance of a violation, during which time the product cannot be distributed.

In other circumstances, when the agency identifies a food product with labeling that is false or misleading (misbranded), it may inform the manufacturer, often in the form of a warning letter, of the violation of law and ask the firm to correct the problem. Most firms contacted by FDA about a labeling violation voluntarily comply, Roosevelt says.

Those that do not can be subject to additional legal action to remove the misbranded products from commerce. Under such circumstances, these products cannot return to the market until the manufacturers take action to correct the violations.

"In the case of the pomegranate juice," Roosevelt says, "the burden is on the importer to show that the product labeling is accurate." "Otherwise, the juice is not going to make it into the U.S."

Another example: In 2012, FDA issued an import alert for shipments of honey exported from India, Malaysia, New Zealand, Turkey and Vietnam due to findings that certain honey products from these countries had been adulterated through the partial substitution of cane or corn sweeteners.

Import alerts are listed on fda.gov, and there are a number of different ways to search for firms and products. FDA also maintains an alphabetical list of warning letters by subject in which consumers can find previous examples of past warning letters citing misbranding or adulteration of food.

Regulations Set Standards

In addition, FDA regulations include formal standards of identity for many kinds of food, including milk and cream; cheese and related cheese products; frozen desserts; bakery products; cereal flours and related products; macaroni and noodle products; canned fruits; canned fruit juices; fruit butters, jellies, preserves and related products; fruit pies; canned vegetables; vegetable juices; frozen vegetables; eggs and egg products; fish and shellfish; cacao products, tree nut and peanut products; beverages; margarine; sweeteners and table syrups; and food dressings and flavorings.

These regulations help to protect consumers against the intentional substitution of ingredients without declaring those ingredients in labeling (e.g., using an unlisted, less expensive ingredient to reduce the cost of manufacturing). The standards of identity require that products contain the ingredients required by the standard.

"In other words," says Roosevelt, "the product is what the label says it is."

What A Consumer Can Do

Each year, millions of Americans have allergic reactions to food. Although most food allergies cause relatively mild and minor symptoms, some food allergies can cause severe reactions, and may even be life threatening.

There is no cure for food allergies. Strict avoidance of food allergens—and early recognition and management of allergic reactions to food—are important measures to prevent serious health consequences.

(Source: "Food Allergens," U.S. Food and Drug Administration (FDA).)

FDA receives much of its information on possible product labeling violations from competitors in industry, at which point the agency often examines or tests the product to confirm or disprove the claims.

If consumers suspect a label is inaccurate, however, FDA welcomes information from them as well. Consumer complaint coordinators located in 19 FDA district offices throughout the United States and Puerto Rico will listen, document your complaint or concern, and determine the appropriate contact for follow-up. You can find the number of the complaint coordinator in your area.

Chapter 56

The Food Allergen Labeling and Consumer Protection Act (FALCPA)

The Food Allergen Labeling and Consumer Protection Act (FALCPA) of 2004 is an amendment to the Federal Food, Drug, and Cosmetic Act (FD&C Act) and requires that the label of a food that contains an ingredient that is or contains protein from a "major food allergen" declare the presence of the allergen in the manner described by the law.

FAQs On FALCPA

Why Did Congress Pass This Act?

Congress passed this Act to make it easier for food allergic consumers and their caregivers to identify and avoid foods that contain major food allergens. In fact, in a review of the foods of randomly selected manufacturers of baked goods, ice cream, and candy in Minnesota and Wisconsin in 1999, The U.S. Food and Drug Administration (FDA) found that 25 percent of sampled foods failed to list peanuts or eggs as ingredients on the food labels although the foods contained these allergens.

When Did FALCPA Become Effective?

FALCPA applies to food products that are labeled on or after January 1, 2006.

About This Chapter: This chapter includes text excerpted from "Food Allergen Labeling And Consumer Protection Act Of 2004 Questions And Answers," U.S. Food and Drug Administration (FDA), November 30, 2016.

What Is A "Major Food Allergen?"

FALCPA identifies eight foods or food groups as the major food allergens. They are milk, eggs, fish (e.g., bass, flounder, cod), Crustacean shellfish (e.g., crab, lobster, shrimp), tree nuts (e.g., almonds, walnuts, pecans), peanuts, wheat, and soybeans.

FALCPA Identifies Only 8 Allergens. Aren't There More Foods Consumers Are Allergic To?

Yes. More than 160 foods have been identified to cause food allergies in sensitive individuals. However, the eight major food allergens identified by FALCPA account for over 90 percent of all documented food allergies in the United States and represent the foods most likely to result in severe or life-threatening reactions.

How Serious Are Food Allergies?

It is estimated that 2 percent of adults and about 5 percent of infants and young children in the United States suffer from food allergies. Approximately 30,000 consumers require emergency room treatment and 150 Americans die each year because of allergic reactions to food.

Does FALCPA Apply To Imported Foods As Well?

FALCPA applies to both domestically manufactured and imported packaged foods that are subject to FDA regulation.

Will FDA Establish A Threshold Level For Any Allergen?

FDA may consider a threshold level for one or more food allergens.

How Will Food Labels Change As A Result Of FALCPA?

FALCPA requires food manufacturers to label food products that contain an ingredient that is or contains protein from a major food allergen in one of two ways.

The first option for food manufacturers is to include the name of the food source in parenthesis following the common or usual name of the major food allergen in the list of ingredients in instances when the name of the food source of the major allergen does not appear elsewhere in the ingredient statement.

The second option is to place the word "Contains" followed by the name of the food source from which the major food allergen is derived, immediately after or adjacent to the list of ingredients, in type size that is no smaller than the type size used for the list of ingredients. For example: Contains Wheat, Milk, Egg, and Soy.

Will The Ingredient List Be Specific About What Type Of Tree Nut, Fish, Or Shellfish Is In The Product?

FALCPA requires the type of tree nut (e.g., almonds, pecans, walnuts); the type of fish (e.g., bass, flounder, cod); and the type of Crustacean shellfish (e.g., crab, lobster, shrimp) to be declared.

Does FALCPA Require The Use Of A "May Contain" Statement In Any Circumstance?

No. Advisory statements are not required by FALCPA.

Are Flavors, Colors, And Food Additives Subject To The Allergen Labeling Requirements?

Yes. FALCPA requires that food manufacturers label food products that contain ingredients, including a flavoring, coloring, or incidental additive that are, or contain, a major food allergen using plain English to identify the allergens.

Are There Any Foods Exempt From The New Labeling Requirements?

Yes. Under FALCPA, raw agricultural commodities (generally fresh fruits and vegetables) are exempt as are highly refined oils derived from one of the eight major food allergens and any ingredient derived from such highly refined oil.

Can Food Manufacturers Ask To Have A Product Exempted From The New Labeling Requirements?

Yes. FALCPA provides mechanisms by which a manufacturer may request that a food ingredient covered by FALCPA may be exempt from FALCPA's labeling requirements. An ingredient may be exempt if it does not cause an allergic response that poses a risk to human health or if it does not contain allergenic protein.

What Does FDA Require In Order For A Product To Be Exempt?

FALCPA states that any person can petition the Secretary of Health and Human Services for an exemption either through a petition process or a notification process.

The petition process requires scientific evidence (including the analytical method used to produce the evidence) that demonstrates that such food ingredient, as derived by the method specified in the petition, does not cause an allergic response that poses a risk to human health.

The notification process must include scientific evidence (including the analytical method used) that demonstrates that the food ingredient (as derived by the production method specified in the notification) does not contain allergenic protein.

If either the petition or the notification is granted by the Secretary, the result is that the ingredient in question is not considered a "major food allergen" and is not subject to the labeling requirements.

For a list of the notifications for exemptions FDA has received, see: Inventory of Notifications Received under 21 U.S.C. 343(w)(7) for Exemptions from Food Allergen Labeling; for a list of the petitions for exemptions FDA has received, see: Inventory of Petitions Received under 21 U.S.C. 343(w)(6) for Exemptions from Food Allergen Labeling.

How Will FDA Make Sure Food Manufacturers Adhere To The New Labeling Regulations?

As a part of its routine regulatory functions, FDA inspects a variety of packaged foods to ensure that they are properly labeled.

What Is Cross Contact?

Cross contact is the inadvertent introduction of an allergen into a product. It is generally the result of environmental exposure during processing or handling, which may occur when multiple foods are produced in the same facility. It may occur due to use of the same processing line, through the misuse of rework, as the result of ineffective cleaning, or from the generation of dust or aerosols containing an allergen.

Why Is There A Concern About Gluten?

Gluten describes a group of proteins found in certain grains (wheat, barley, and rye.) It is of concern because people with celiac disease cannot tolerate it. Celiac disease (also known as celiac sprue) is a chronic digestive disease that damages the small intestine and interferes with absorption of nutrients from food. Recent findings estimate that 2 million people in the United States have celiac disease or about 1 in 133 people.

How Can I Avoid Foods To Which I'm Allergic?

FDA advises consumers to work with healthcare providers to find out what food(s) can cause an allergic reaction. In addition, consumers who are allergic to major food allergens should read the ingredient statement on food products to determine if products contain a major allergen. A "Contains_____" statement, if present on a label, can also be used to determine if the food contains a major food allergen.

But I Don't Understand What Some Of The Terms Mean. How Will I Know What They Are?

FALCPA was designed to improve food labeling information so that consumers who suffer from food allergies, especially children and their caregivers will be able to recognize the presence of an ingredient that they must avoid. For example, if a product contains the milk derived protein casein, the product's label would have to use the term "milk" in addition to the term "casein" so that those with milk allergies would clearly understand the presence of an allergen they need to avoid.

What About Food Prepared In Restaurants? How Will I Know That The Food I Ordered Does Not Contain An Ingredient To Which I Am Allergic?

FALCPA only applies to packaged FDA regulated foods. However, FDA advises consumers who are allergic to particular foods to ask questions about ingredients and preparation when eating at restaurants or any place outside the consumer's home.

How Will FALCPA Apply To Foods Purchased At Bakeries, Food Kiosks At The Mall, And Carry Out Restaurants?

FALCPA's labeling requirements extend to retail and food service establishments that package, label, and offer products for human consumption. However, FALCPA's labeling requirements do not apply to foods that are placed in a wrapper or container in response to a consumer's order such as the paper or box used to provide a sandwich ordered by a consumer.

Chapter 57

Going Out To Eat With Food Allergies

Rick, Lois, Angus, and Samantha visit a new restaurant to celebrate Rick's birthday. They are excited to try the restaurant they've heard so much about. The host seats them and they start looking over their menus to decide what to order. Lois is allergic to peanuts, so she wonders about the ingredients in the eggrolls.

The server approaches the table to take their orders. Lois asks if the restaurant has an ingredient list for the egg rolls. The server says yes and brings the list. Lois sees that the eggrolls contain peanuts, but the salad doesn't, so she decides to have the salad instead.

Rick and his friends enjoy their meal and say they want to eat there again and try something else from the menu.

Before the restaurant opened last month, staff received training on food allergies including what to do if a customer has an allergic reaction. The food safety certified kitchen manager also prepared ingredient lists for all menu items, and the kitchen has dedicated areas and equipment for preparing and cooking food for customers with food allergies.

Food allergies are a growing public health issue—about 15 million Americans have food allergies. And food allergic reactions are responsible for about 30,000 emergency room visits and 150–200 deaths a year.

Many food allergic reactions occur in restaurants. One in three people with food allergies have had a reaction in a restaurant. Understanding how restaurants address food allergies can help to reduce the risk of food allergic reactions in restaurants.

About This Chapter: This chapter includes text excerpted from "Going Out To Eat with Food Allergies," Centers for Disease Control and Prevention (CDC), May 17, 2017.

How Restaurants Address Food Allergies

Key Findings And Recommendations

Most restaurants could do more to reduce the risk of food allergic reactions.

- Less than half of interviewed restaurant staff had received training on food allergies. And training often didn't cover important information such as what to do if a customer has an allergic reaction.

- Most restaurants did not have dedicated areas and equipment for preparing and cooking allergen-free food.

Most restaurants did have ingredient lists or recipes for some or all of their menu items. Ingredient lists and recipes are important tools in reducing the risk of food allergic reactions. Customers with food allergies rely on restaurant staff to provide them with accurate information on ingredients.

It's recommended that restaurants

- Provide food allergy training for staff.

- Use dedicated equipment and areas for preparing and cooking meals for customers with food allergies. When this is not feasible, restaurants can clean equipment and workspaces before preparing meals for customers with allergies, according to the U.S. Food and Drug Administration's (FDA) Food Code guidance.

- Have ingredient lists or recipes for menu items available if they aren't already.

These practices can help reduce the risk of an allergic reaction.

Study Problem

Food allergies are a growing public health issue:

- About 15 million Americans have food allergies.

- Food allergic reactions are responsible for about 30,000 emergency room visits and 150–200 deaths a year.

Many food allergic reactions occur in restaurants—one in three people with food allergies have had a reaction in a restaurant. Understanding how restaurants address food allergies can help to reduce the risk of food allergic reactions in restaurants.

Study Purpose

The purpose of this study was to find out how many restaurants

- Train their staff on food allergies.

- Have ingredient lists and special equipment and areas for making food for customers with food allergies.

Study Results

Less than half of interviewed restaurant staff had been trained on food allergies.

In 4 of 5 restaurants, food allergy training covered:

- How to prevent cross-contact.

- The major food allergens.

- What to do if a customer has a food allergy.

In 3 of 5 restaurants, food allergy training covered:

- Symptoms of an allergic reaction.

- What to do if someone has an allergic reaction.

Most restaurants had ingredient lists or recipes for some or all menu items. But few restaurants had dedicated equipment and areas for preparing and cooking allergen-free food.

Chapter 58

Food Allergy Lab Fits On Your Keychain

More than 50 million Americans have food allergies and often just trace amounts of allergens can trigger life-threatening reactions. Now, National Institute of Biomedical Imaging and Bioengineering (NIBIB)-funded researchers at Harvard Medical School have developed a $40 device that fits on a key chain and can accurately test for allergens, like gluten or nuts, in a restaurant meal in less than 10 minutes.

Food allergies are extremely common. Those fortunate enough not to be affected are likely to have a friend or family member who struggles to avoid dangerous reactions to food allergens every day. In the United States, Federal regulations require packaged foods to disclose the presence of some of the most common allergens such as gluten, nuts, and milk products, which is helpful, but not always accurate.

When it comes to eating out, people with allergies have had to rely on their knowledge of what ingredients contain the allergens they must avoid, and on the efforts of the restaurant to provide dishes that eliminate allergens; and they must work to avoid cross-contamination between different ingredients in the kitchen. All in all, this approach generally leaves those with allergies with little choice but to completely avoid any foods that have the chance of containing an allergen, either in the natural ingredients, or because of contact with other foods containing allergens during preparation in a restaurant kitchen.

About This Chapter: This chapter includes text excerpted from "Food Allergy Lab Fits On Your Keychain," National Institute of Biomedical Imaging and Bioengineering (NIBIB), October 25, 2017.

Individuals With Allergies Can Test Their Meal At The Restaurant Table

Recognizing this widespread public health problem, researchers at Harvard Medical School in Boston have developed a system called integrated exogenous antigen testing (iEAT). The purpose of the iEAT system is to give those who suffer from food allergies a rapid, accurate device that allows them to personally test foods in less than 10 minutes.

Development of the iEAT system was led by co-senior team leaders Ralph Weissleder, M.D., Ph.D., the Thrall Professor of Radiology, Professor of Systems Biology at Harvard, and Director of the Center for Systems Biology (CSB) at Massachusetts General Hospital (MGH); and Hakho Lee, Ph.D., Associate Professor in Radiology at Harvard, Hostetter MGH Research Scholar, and Director of the Biomedical Engineering Program at the CSB, MGH. The work, is published in the August 2017 issue of *ACS Nano*.

"This invention is a fortuitous combination of the interests and expertise of Drs. Weissleder and Lee in developing tools for early disease detection, magnetic sensors, and point-of-care diagnostics," said Shumin Wang, Ph.D., director of the NIBIB program in Biomagnetic and Bioelectric Devices. "They have taken technologies they developed for other medical problems, such as early cancer detection from blood samples, and applied them to solving the daily, potentially life-threatening difficulties of people with food allergies—a highly significant public health problem that incurs 25 billion dollars in annual costs in the United States alone."

The device consists of three components. A small plastic test tube is used to dissolve a small sample of the food being tested and to add the magnetic beads that capture the food allergen of interest, such as gluten. A bit of that solution is then dropped onto electrode strips on a small module that is then inserted into the electronic keychain reader. The keychain reader has a small display that indicates whether the allergen is present, and if so, in what concentration. Testing showed that measurements of the concentration of the allergen is extremely accurate.

The high level of accuracy is very important. For example, even though Federal standards say that a food is considered gluten free if it has a concentration of less than 20 mg per kg of gluten, everyone's sensitivity is different, and many people would have a reaction at much lower gluten concentrations. Extensive testing of iEAT revealed that the system could detect levels of gluten that were 200 times lower than the Federal standard.

"High accuracy built into a compact system were the key goals of the project," says Weissleder. "Users can be confident that even if they are sensitive to very low levels, iEAT will be able to give them exact concentrations. Armed with accurate concentration levels they will not have to completely avoid potentially problematic foods, but will know whether an allergen is at a dangerous level for them or a concentration that is safe for them to eat."

Beyond obtaining the information they need in about 10 minutes using iEAT, a novel addition to the system was the development of a cell phone app, which offers the possibility of addressing food allergies at the community level. Using the app, users can compile and store the data they collect as they test different foods for various allergens at different restaurants and even in packaged foods. The app is set up to share this information online with both time and location stamps indicating when, where, and in what food or dish an allergen reading was taken. With the app, people will eventually have a personal record of levels that trigger a reaction. Others with the app will be able to find restaurants with foods they like to eat that consistently have no or low levels that are below the individual's triggering concentration.

"Although we believed iEAT could address a significant public health problem, we were surprised at the amount of interest the device has generated. We are receiving calls from people asking if we can adapt iEAT to test for other substances such as MSG or even pesticides," said Hakho Lee, co-senior leader of the project. "The good news is that we definitely can adapt the device to test for just about any allergen or substance."

Towards that end, the research team has granted a license to a local start-up company to make iEAT commercially available. The company plans to merge the three components into a single module to make it even easier and more convenient to use. Production on a larger scale is also expected to reduce the price of the unit considerably.

In addition to contributing to food safety at the individual and community levels in the United States, the inventors point out that the device would be very valuable for travelers in countries where there are no specific requirements for food labels. Another use of the system would be to trace the source of food contamination with bacteria such as *E. Coli* or *Salmonella* to a specific food-processing site by testing DNA in the samples to potentially identify and contain an outbreak more quickly.

Chapter 59

Working With A Dietitian

Learning that a child has food allergies can be frightening for parents. Once an allergist has diagnosed food allergies, many parents feel overwhelmed by the challenge of eliminating allergenic foods while also providing their child with healthy, nutritious meals. Without proper meal planning and supplementation, the dietary restrictions caused by food allergies can affect nutrient intake and potentially harm a child's growth, development, and future health.

Up to 90 percent of food-related allergic reactions in the United States can be traced to eight foods: cow's milk, eggs, wheat, soy, peanuts, tree nuts, fish, and shellfish. Yet these foods are high in vitamins, minerals, and other important nutrients. Nuts, for instance, are rich in vitamin E, niacin, manganese, magnesium, and chromium. As a result, at least 25 percent of children with food allergies experience vitamin and mineral deficiencies.

When certain foods must be eliminated from a child's diet, parents need to find ways to replace the nutrients that they provide. Many parents find it helpful to work with a registered dietitian in order to create meal plans that are appetizing and nutritious while also eliminating allergens. Dietitians can help ease parental anxiety by providing individualized education about how to avoid certain foods and substitute safe alternatives. They can also help families ensure that the child with food allergies receives adequate nutrition to promote growth and development. Finally, a registered dietitian can devise an action plan to help families cope with situations in which the child might encounter allergens.

About This Chapter: "Working With A Dietitian," © 2016 Omnigraphics. Reviewed November 2017.

Dietitians and nutritionists are experts in the use of food and nutrition to promote health and manage disease. They advise people on what to eat in order to lead a healthy lifestyle or achieve a specific health-related goal.

Dietitians and nutritionists work in many settings, including hospitals, nursing homes, clinics, cafeterias, and for state and local governments.

Dietitians and nutritionists typically need a bachelor's degree, along with supervised training through an internship. Many states require dietitians and nutritionists to be licensed.

(Source: "Dietitians And Nutritionists," Bureau of Labor Statistics (BLS).)

Choosing A Qualified Dietitian

Training for dietitians in the United States includes four years of college to obtain a bachelor's degree in nutrition and dietetics, followed by a stipulated period of internship or professional practice. Dietitians are also required to pass a registration examination conducted by the Commission on Dietetic Registration before they can become a Registered Dietitian (RD). Many dietitians specialize in certain areas by working under other professional dietitians. They also keep abreast with the latest developments in the field by attending seminars and workshops regularly.

Parents of children with food allergies who are interested in working with a dietitian should first assess the person's qualifications and experience. Experts advise asking prospective dietitians about their education, training, and professional memberships. It may also be helpful to know how long they have treated patients with food allergies and what specialized training they have undertaken to gain proficiency in treating food allergies. The American Dietetic Association (ADA) maintains a searchable list of registered dietitians on its website, www.eatright.org.

How The Dietitian Can Help

During the initial consultation with parents of a child with food allergies, a dietitian is likely to ask what the child eats on a regular basis, what foods have been identified as allergens, and what symptoms the child has experienced. This information will help the dietitian develop a meal plan for the child that includes safe alternative foods and provides all the nutrients the child needs to grow and thrive. The dietitian's goal is to provide suggestions for healthy, nutritious meals that offer a variety of food choices that the child will enjoy.

The dietitian can also provide parents with expert advice on how to avoid allergenic foods, from reading product labels to recognizing places where cross-contamination or accidental exposure could occur—such as school classrooms, restaurants, movie theaters, or airplanes. The dietitian can also give parents an extensive list of safe alternatives that they can substitute for allergy-inducing foods in meals or recipes.

Many dietitians ask families to keep a diary of the child's daily meals—noting any allergy symptoms observed—in order to facilitate meal planning. The dietitian will also monitor the child's growth and development through regular follow-up sessions and suggest dietary changes over time to meet their nutritional needs. Since children often outgrow allergies to certain foods, the dietitian can watch for these changes and help parents reintroduce the foods in a gradual and safe manner.

References

1. Bowers, Elizabeth Shimer. "Can a Dietitian Help with Children's Food Allergies?" Everyday Health, May 27, 2015.

2. Feuling, Mary Beth. "The Balancing Act: Nutrition and Food Allergy." Children's Hospital of Wisconsin, October 2015.

Chapter 60

A Food Diary Can Reduce Risk Of Reactions

Food allergies have emerged as a growing health crisis. They affect 15 million people in the United States, including 4 percent of adults and 8 percent of children, and account for 200,000 emergency room visits per year. When someone develops a food allergy, the body's immune system overreacts to the allergenic food by releasing histamines and other chemicals into the bloodstream. This process can cause a number of different symptoms to occur, such as hives, rashes, nasal congestion, breathing difficulties, diarrhea, nausea, and vomiting. Although some people experience only minor symptoms, food allergies can also trigger anaphylaxis, a severe, whole-body allergic reaction that is potentially fatal.

It is not always easy to identify which food can trigger an allergic reaction. For some people the symptoms could be obviously related to a particular food, and for others the symptoms could appear mysteriously, making the allergen difficult to pinpoint. Not even diagnostic tests conducted by experts can precisely recognize food allergens in all cases. To help people identify the cause and manage their food allergy on an everyday basis, one of the best methods is to keep a written record of everything they eat.

Keeping A Food Diary

A food journal should be maintained on an everyday basis and record the details of every meal, beverage, snack, and dietary supplement. In addition, each entry should include any noticeable symptoms after a meal, even just a general feeling of indigestion or fatigue. The details that should be noted in the food diary include the symptoms experienced, whether

About This Chapter: "A Food Diary Can Reduce Risk Of Reactions," © 2016 Omnigraphics. Reviewed November 2017.

they were mild or severe, and their duration. Other information that could be included in the journal include any medications taken; any exposure to environmental allergens such as pollen, dust mites, mold, perfumes, latex, or pet dander; any other illnesses or conditions experienced, such as the common cold, hepatitis, and insect bites; and any symptoms that were a result of physical stimuli, such as heat, cold, pressure, exercise, and extreme sun exposure.

It is important to note that a food item may contain a number of ingredients. Any kind of ingredient may cause an allergic reaction, which could range from mild to severe. If the symptoms occur while eating in a place other than home—for instance, at a restaurant—it would be helpful to talk to the chef and ask for a list of all the ingredients used in the food consumed.

If the allergic reaction is due to processed or prepackaged food, the label should be saved and the quantity consumed should be noted.

All the information noted in the food diary can help an allergist make an informed diagnosis of the cause of allergy symptoms and determine the best course of treatment. A number of helpful food journal applications are available for mobile phone and tablet users to keep track of their allergies. Identifying and avoiding food culprits can help people maintain their health wisely and enjoy a better quality of life.

Reference

"Identifying Your Food Intolerances," Allergy UK, October 2012.

Chapter 61

Egg Allergies And Vaccines

What Is Considered An Egg Allergy? What Are The Signs And Symptoms Of An Egg Allergic Reaction?

Egg allergy can be confirmed by a consistent medical history of adverse reactions to eggs and egg-containing foods, plus skin, and/or blood testing for immunoglobulin E (IgE) antibodies to egg proteins. Persons who are able to eat lightly cooked egg (e.g., scrambled egg) without reaction are unlikely to be allergic. Egg-allergic persons might tolerate egg in baked products (e.g., bread or cake). Therefore, tolerance to egg-containing foods does not exclude the possibility of egg allergy. Egg allergies can range in severity.

How Common Is Egg Allergy In Children And Adults?

Egg allergy affects about 1.3 percent of all children and 0.2 percent of all adults.

What Vaccine Should I Get If I Am Egg Allergic, But I Can Eat Lightly Cooked Eggs?

If you are able to eat lightly cooked egg (e.g., scrambled egg) without reaction, you are unlikely to be allergic and can get any licensed flu vaccine (i.e., any form of IIV, LAIV, or RIV) that is otherwise appropriate for your age and health status.

About This Chapter: This chapter includes text excerpted from "Seasonal Influenza (Flu)—Flu Vaccine And People With Egg Allergies," Centers for Disease Control and Prevention (CDC), September 2, 2016.

What Flu Vaccine Should I Get If I Get Hives After Eating Egg-Containing Foods?

If you are someone with a history of egg allergy, who has experienced only hives after exposure to egg, you can get any licensed flu vaccine (i.e., any form of IIV, LAIV, or RIV) that is otherwise appropriate for your age and health.

What Kind Of Flu Vaccine Should I Get If I Have More Serious Reactions To Eating Eggs Or Egg-Containing Foods Like Cardiovascular Changes Or A Reaction Requiring Epinephrine?

If you are someone who has more serious reactions to eating eggs or egg-containing foods, like angioedema, respiratory distress, lightheadedness, or recurrent emesis; or who required epinephrine or another emergency medical intervention, you can get any licensed flu vaccine (i.e., any form of IIV, LAIV, or RIV) that is otherwise appropriate for your age and health status, but the vaccine should be given by a healthcare provider who can recognize and respond to a severe allergic response.

Are There Still People With Egg Allergies Who Should Not Get Flu Vaccine?

People with egg allergy can receive flu vaccines according to the recommendations above. A person who has previously experienced a severe allergic reaction to flu vaccine, regardless of the component suspected of being responsible for the reaction should not get a flu vaccine again.

Why Do Flu Vaccines Contain Egg Protein?

Most flu vaccines today are produced using an egg-based manufacturing process and thus contain a small amount of egg protein called ovalbumin.

How Much Egg Protein Is In Flu Vaccine?

While not all manufacturers disclose the amount of ovalbumin in their vaccines, those that did from 2011–12 through 2014–15 reported maximum amounts of ≤1 µg/0.5 mL dose for flu shots and 0.24 µg/0.2 mL dose for the nasal spray vaccine. Cell-based flu vaccine (Flucelvax) likely has a much smaller amount of egg protein since the original vaccine virus is grown in eggs, but mass production of that vaccine does not occur in eggs. Recombinant vaccine (Flublok) is the only vaccine currently available that is completely egg free.

Can Egg Protein In Flu Vaccine Cause Allergic Reactions In Persons With A History Of Egg Allergy?

Yes, allergic reactions can happen, but they occur very rarely with the flu vaccines available in the United States today. Occasional cases of anaphylaxis, a severe life-threatening reaction that involves multiple organ systems and can progress rapidly, in egg-allergic persons have been reported to the Vaccine Adverse Event Reporting System (VAERS) after administration of flu vaccine. Flu vaccines contain various components that may cause allergic reactions, including anaphylaxis. In a Vaccine Safety Datalink (VSD) study, there were 10 cases of anaphylaxis after more than 7.4 million doses of inactivated flu vaccine, trivalent (IIV3) given without other vaccines, (rate of 1.35 per one million doses). Most of these cases of anaphylaxis were not related to the egg protein present in the vaccine. Centers for Disease Control and Prevention (CDC) and the Advisory Committee on Immunization Practices (ACIP) continue to review available data regarding anaphylaxis cases following flu vaccines.

How Long After Flu Vaccination Does A Reaction Occur In Persons With A History Of Egg Allergy?

Allergic reactions can begin very soon after vaccination. However, the onset of symptoms is sometimes delayed. In a VSD study of more than 25.1 million doses of vaccines of various types given to children and adults over 3 years, only 33 people had anaphylaxis. Of patients with a documented time to onset of symptoms, eight cases had onset within 30 minutes of vaccination, while in another 21 cases, symptoms were delayed more than 30 minutes following vaccination, including one case with symptom onset on the following day.

CDC Recommendations for 2016–2017

Centers for Disease Control and Prevention (CDC) and its Advisory Committee on Immunization Practices have updated their guidelines on egg allergy and receipt of influenza (flu) vaccines. Based on the new recommendations, people with egg allergies no longer need to be observed for an allergic reaction for 30 minutes after receiving a flu vaccine. Should it be required, people with a history of severe allergic reaction to egg (i.e., any symptom other than hives) can now be vaccinated in an inpatient or outpatient medical setting (including but not necessarily limited to hospitals, clinics, health departments, and physician offices), under the supervision of any healthcare provider who is able to recognize and manage severe allergic conditions. Previously, it was recommended that such people be given a flu vaccine only by a doctor with experience in managing severe allergic conditions and that they be observed for 30 minutes after vaccination.

Most flu shots and the nasal spray flu vaccine are manufactured using egg-based technology. Because of this, they contain a small amount of egg proteins, such as ovalbumin. However, studies that have examined the use of both the nasal spray vaccine and flu shots in egg-allergic and nonegg-allergic patients indicate that severe allergic reactions in people with egg allergies are unlikely. A CDC study found the rate of anaphylaxis after all vaccines is 1.31 per one million vaccine doses given.

Part Six
If You Need More Information

Chapter 62

Resources For Allergy Information

Government Agencies That Provide Information About Allergy

Agency for Healthcare Research and Quality (AHRQ)
Office of Communications and Knowledge Transfer
5600 Fishers Ln.
Seventh Fl.
Rockville, MD 20857
Phone: 301-427-1364
Website: www.ahrq.gov

Center for Food Safety and Applied Nutrition (CFSAN)
U.S. Food and Drug Administration (FDA)
5001 Campus Dr.
HFS-009
College Park, MD 20740-3835
Toll-Free: 888-SAFEFOOD (888-723-3366)
Website: www.fda.gov/food

About This Chapter: Resources in this chapter were compiled from several sources deemed reliable; all contact information was verified and updated in November 2017.

Centers for Disease Control and Prevention (CDC)
1600 Clifton Rd.
Atlanta, GA 30329-4027
Toll-Free: 800-CDC-INFO (800-232-4636)
Phone: 404-639-3311
Toll-Free TTY: 888-232-6348
Website: www.cdc.gov

Healthfinder®
National Health Information Center (NHIC)
1101 Wootton Pkwy
Rockville, MD 20852
Website: www.healthfinder.gov
E-mail: healthfinder@hhs.gov

National Center for Complementary and Integrative Health (NCCIH)
9000 Rockville Pike
Bethesda, MD 20892
Toll-Free: 888-644-6226
Toll-Free TTY: 866-464-3615
Toll-Free Fax: 866-464-3616
Website: www.nccih.nih.gov
E-mail: info@nccih.nih.gov

National Center for Environmental Health (NCEH)
Centers for Disease Control and Prevention (CDC)
4770 Buford Hwy N.E.
Atlanta, GA 30341-3717
Toll-Free: 800-232-4636
Phone: 404-639-2520
Toll-Free TTY: 888-232-6348
Website: www.cdc.gov/nceh
E-mail: cdcinfo@cdc.gov

National Digestive Diseases Information Clearinghouse (NDDIC)
Toll-Free: 800-860-8747
Toll-Free TTY: 866-569-1162
Fax: 703-738-4929
Website: www.niddk.nih.gov/health-information/digestive-diseases
E-mail: healthinfo@niddk.nih.gov

National Heart, Lung, and Blood Institute (NHLBI)

Bldg. 31 Rm. 5A52
31 Center Dr. MSC 2486
Bethesda, MD 20892
Phone: 301-592-8573
TTY: 240-629-3255
Fax: 301-629-3246
Website: www.nhlbi.nih.gov
E-mail: nhlbiinfo@nhlbi.nih.gov

National Institute of Allergy and Infectious Diseases (NIAID)

5601 Fishers Ln.
MSC 9806
Bethesda, MD 20892-9806
Toll-Free: 866-284-4107
Phone: 301-496-5717
TDD: 800-877-8339
Fax: 301-402-3573
Website: www.niaid.nih.gov
E-mail: ocpostoffice@niaid.nih.gov

National Institute of Arthritis and Musculoskeletal and Skin Diseases (NIAMS)

Bldg. 31 Rm. 4C02
31 Center Dr. MSC 2350
Bethesda, MD 20892-2350
Toll-Free: 877-22-NIAMS (877-226-4267)
Phone: 301-496-8190
TTY: 301–565–2966
Fax: 301-480-2814
Website: www.niams.nih.gov
E-mail: niamsinfo@mail.nih.gov

National Institute of Diabetes and Digestive and Kidney Diseases (NIDDK)

31 Center Dr. MSC 2560
Bldg. 31 Rm. 9A06
Bethesda, MD 20892-2560
Phone: 301-496-3583
Website: www.niddk.nih.gov

National Institute of Environmental Health Sciences (NIEHS)
111 T.W. Alexander Dr.
Durham, NC 27709
Phone: 919-541-3345
Fax: 301-480-2978
Website: www.niehs.nih.gov
E-mail: webcenter@niehs.nih.gov

National Institutes of Health (NIH)
9000 Rockville Pike
Bethesda, MD 20892
Phone: 301-496-4000
Website: www.nih.gov
E-mail: NIHinfo@od.nih.gov

U.S. Department of Agriculture (USDA)
1400 Independence Ave. S.W.
Washington, DC 20250
Phone: 202-720-2791
Website: www.usda.gov

U.S. Environmental Protection Agency (EPA)
1200 Pennsylvania Ave. N.W.
Washington, DC 20460
Phone: 202-564-4700
TTY: 202-272-0165
Website: www.epa.gov

U.S. Food and Drug Administration (FDA)
10903 New Hampshire Ave.
Silver Spring, MD 20993
Toll-Free: 888-INFO-FDA (888-463-6332)
Website: www.fda.gov

U.S. National Library of Medicine (NLM)
8600 Rockville Pike
Bethesda, MD 20894
Toll-Free: 888-FIND-NLM (888-346-3656)
Toll-Free TDD: 800-735-2258
Fax: 301-402-1384
Website: www.nlm.nih.gov
E-mail: custserv@nlm.nih.gov

Private Agencies That Provide Information About Allergy

Academy of Nutrition and Dietetics
120 S. Riverside Plaza
Ste. 2190
Chicago, IL 60606-6995
Toll-Free: 800-877-1600
Phone: 312-899-0040
Website: www.eatright.org
E-mail: acend@eatright.org

Allergic Living Magazine
P.O. Box 1042
Niagara Falls, NY 14304
Toll-Free: 888-771-7747
Phone: 416-604-0110
Website: www.allergicliving.com
E-mail: info@allergicliving.com

AllergicChild.com
6660 Delmonico Dr.
Ste. D249
Colorado Springs, CO 80919
Website: www.allergicchild.com

Allergy and Asthma Information Association (AAIA)

200-5409 Eglinton Ave. W.
Toronto, ON M9C 5K6
Canada
Toll-Free: 800-611-7011
Phone: 416-621-4571
Fax: 416-621-5034
Website: www.aaia.ca
E-mail: admin@aaia.ca

Allergy and Asthma Network Mothers of Asthmatics (AANMA)

8229 Boone Blvd.
Ste. 260
Vienna, VA 22182
Toll-Free: 800-878-4403
Fax: 703-288-5271
Website: www.allergyasthmanetwork.org

Allergy UK

Planwell House
LEFA Business Park
Edgington Way
Sidcup, Kent DA14 5BH
United Kingdom
Phone: +44 0 13 22 619898
Website: www.allergyuk.org
E-mail: info@allergyuk.org

American Academy of Allergy, Asthma and Immunology (AAAAI)

555 E. Wells St.
Ste. 1100
Milwaukee, WI 53202-3823
Phone: 414-272-6071
Website: www.aaaai.org
E-mail: info@aaaai.org

American Academy of Dermatology (AAD)
930 E. Woodfield Rd.
Schaumburg, IL 60173
Toll-Free: 866-503-SKIN (866-503-7546)
Phone: 847-240-1280
Fax: 847-240-1859
Website: www.aad.org
E-mail: mrc@aad.org

American Academy of Otolaryngology-Head and Neck Surgery (AAO-HNS)
1650 Diagonal Rd.
Alexandria, VA 22314-2857
Phone: 703-836-4444
Website: www.entnet.org

American Board of Allergy and Immunology (ABAI)
1835 Market St.
Ste. 1210
Philadelphia, PA 19103
Toll-Free: 866-264-5568
Phone: 215-592-9466
Fax: 215-592-9411
Website: www.abai.org
E-mail: abai@abai.org

American College of Allergy, Asthma and Immunology (ACAAI)
85 W. Algonquin Rd.
Ste. 550
Arlington Heights, IL 60005
Phone: 847-427-1200
Fax: 847-427-9656
Website: www.college.acaai.org
E-mail: mail@acaai.org

American Lung Association

55 W. Wacker Dr.
Ste. 1150
Chicago, IL 60601
Toll-Free: 800-LUNGUSA (800-586-4872)
Phone: 312-801-7630
Fax: 202-452-1805
Website: www.lung.org
E-mail: info@lung.org

American Osteopathic College of Dermatology (AOCD)

2902 N. Baltimore St.
P.O. Box 7525
Kirksville, MO 63501
Toll-Free: 800-449-2623
Phone: 660-665-2184
Fax: 660-627-2623
Website: www.aocd.org
E-mail: dermatology@aocd.org

American Partnership for Eosinophilic Disorders (APFED)

P.O. Box 29545
Atlanta, GA 30359
Phone: 713-493-7749
Website: www.apfed.org
E-mail: mail@apfed.org

American Rhinologic Society (ARS)

P.O. Box 269
Oak Ridge, NJ 07438
Phone: 845-988-1631
Fax: 845-986-1527
Website: www.american-rhinologic.org

Asthma and Allergy Foundation of America (AAFA)

8201 Corporate Dr.
Ste. 1000
Landover, MD 20785
Toll-Free: 800-7-ASTHMA (800-727-8462)
Website: www.aafa.org
E-mail: info@aafa.org

Canadian Lung Association

1750 Courtwood Crescent
Ste. 300
Ottawa, ON K2C 2B5
Canada
Toll-Free: 888-566-5864
Phone: 613-569-6411
Fax: 613-569-8860
Website: www.lung.ca
E-mail: info@lung.ca

Celiac Disease Foundation

20350 Ventura Blvd.
Ste. 240
Woodland Hills, CA 91364
Phone: 818-716-1513
Fax: 818-267-5577
Website: www.celiac.org

Food Allergy Canada

2005 Sheppard Ave. E.
Ste. 800
Toronto, ON M2J 5B4
Canada
Toll-Free: 866-785-5660
Phone: 416-785-5666
Fax: 416-785-0458
Toll-Free Fax: 888-872-6014
Website: www.foodallergycanada.ca
E-mail: info@foodallergycanada.ca

Food Allergy Research & Education® (FARE)

7925 Jones Branch Dr.
Ste. 1100
McLean, VA 22102
Toll-Free: 800-929-4040
Phone: 703-691-3179
Fax: 703-691-2713
Website: www.fare.foodallergy.org

Food Allergy Research and Resource Program (FARRP)
University of Nebraska-Lincoln
Rm. 279 Food Innovation Center 1901 N. 21 St.
P.O. Box 886207
Lincoln, NE 68588-6207
Phone: 402-472-7211
Fax: 402-472-5307
Website: www.farrp.unl.edu
E-mail: farrp@unl.edu

International Food Information Council (IFIC)
1100 Connecticut Ave. N.W.
Ste. 430
Washington, DC 20036
Phone: 202-296-6540
Website: www.foodinsight.org
E-mail: info@foodinsight.org

Kids with Food Allergies
4259 W. Swamp Rd.
Ste. 408
Doylestown, PA 18902
Phone: 215-230-5394
Fax: 215-340-7674
Website: www.kidswithfoodallergies.org

National Eczema Association (NEA)
4460 Redwood Hwy
Ste. 16-D
San Rafael, CA 94903
Toll-Free: 800-818-7546
Phone: 415-499-3474
Website: www.nationaleczema.org
E-mail: info@nationaleczema.org

National Jewish Medical and Research Center
1400 Jackson St.
Denver, CO 80206
Toll-Free: 877-CALL-NJH (877-225-5654)
Phone: 303-388-4461
Website: www.nationaljewish.org

Pan American Allergy Society (PAAS)

1317 Wooded Knoll
San Antonio, TX 78258
Phone: 210-495-9853
Fax: 210-495-9852
Website: www.paas.org
E-mail: panamallergy@sbcglobal.net

Pan American Health Organization

525 23rd St. N.W.
Washington, DC 20037
Phone: 202-974-3000
Fax: 202-974-3663
Website: www.paho.org

PeanutAllergy.com

Website: www.peanutallergy.com

Pollen.com

c/o QuintilesIMS
1 IMS Dr.
Plymouth Meeting, PA 19462
Website: www.pollen.com

World Allergy Organization (WAO)

555 E. Wells St.
Ste. 1100
Milwaukee, WI 53202-3823
Phone: 414-276-1791
Fax: 414-276-3349
Website: www.worldallergy.org
E-mail: info@worldallergy.org

Vickerstaff Health Services

2016 High Canada Pl.
Kamloops, BC V2E 2E3
Canada
Phone: 250-377-0945
Fax: 250-377-3248
Website: www.allergynutrition.com
E-mail: vickerstaffhs@allergynutrition.com

Chapter 63

Finding Recipes Online If You Have Food Allergies

Online Recipe Resources For People With Food Allergies

BBC Gluten-Free Recipes
Website: www.bbc.co.uk/food/diets/gluten_free

BBC Nut-Free Recipes
Website: www.bbc.co.uk/food/diets/nut_free

BBC Special Diets Recipes
Website: www.bbcgoodfood.com/recipes/category/special-diets

Cook IT Allergy Free
Website: www.cookitallergyfree.com

Corn-Free Recipes
Website: angelaskitchen.com/recipes/have-other-allergies/corn-free-recipes

Dairy Free Cakes
Website: allrecipes.co.uk/recipes/tag-3191/dairy-free-cake.aspx

Dairy-Free Dinner Recipes
Website: www.bbcgoodfood.com/recipes/collection/dairy-free-dinner

---

About This Chapter: The mobile apps listed in this chapter were compiled from several sources deemed reliable. Inclusion does not constitute endorsement, and there is no implication associated with omission. All website information was verified and updated in November 2017.

Dairy-Free Recipes
Website: www.bbcgoodfood.com/recipes/collection/dairy-free

Eating With Food Allergies
Website: www.eatingwithfoodallergies.com/allergyfreerecipes.html

Egg-Free Recipes
Website: www.bbcgoodfood.com/recipes/collection/egg-free

Food Allergy and Intolerance Self-Diagnosis
Website: www.bbc.com/news/health-17373904

Food Allergy Kitchen
Website: www.foodallergykitchen.co.uk

Food Allergy Research & Education® (FARE): Life With Food Allergies
Website: www.foodallergy.org/life-with-food-allergies

Gluten-Free Cake Recipes
Website: www.bbcgoodfood.com/recipes/collection/gluten-free-cake

Gluten-Free Lunch Recipes
Website: www.bbcgoodfood.com/recipes/collection/gluten-free-lunch

Gluten-Free Snack Recipes
Website: www.bbcgoodfood.com/recipes/collection/gluten-free-snack

Kids With Food Allergies
Website: www.kidswithfoodallergies.com

Living Without
Website: www.livingwithout.com/topics/recipes.html

Peanut Free Recipes
Website: www.peanutallergy.com/nut-free-recipes

20 Tried-and-True Egg-Free Desserts
Website: www.marthastewart.com/1504305/egg-free-desserts

Wheat-Free Recipes
Website: www.wheat-free.org/recipes.html

Mobile Apps Recipe Resources For People With Food Allergies

Allergy Basket
This app helps people keep track of the allergy free foods their family can eat by allowing them to create shopping lists by scanning barcodes.
Website: www.appsforgood.org/public/student-apps/2016/allergy_basket

Allergy Reality: Food Safety
This app is educational gaming app that empowers those with restricted food diets and their loved ones. If you have a food allergy, intolerance, Celiac disease, other autoimmune diseases, or just trying to be conscious of others.
Website: itunes.apple.com/us/app/allergy-reality-food-allergy-learning-and-safety/id1225702477?mt=8

Gluten Free Food Finder
This is a Gluten Free Scanner app that puts users in control of the data. All the data in this app is community sourced. If you disagree with the result of a scan, you can easily change it. If you are the first person to scan an item, please answer a question or two about it.
Website: play.google.com/store/apps/details?id=com.bradclouser.glutenfree&hl=en

iEatOut Gluten Free & Allergy Free
Eat safe ethnic foods using this app. Personalize your food needs with the ethnic restaurant database to confidently avoid gluten, wheat, dairy, egg, peanuts, nuts, soy, corn, fish, and/or shellfish anywhere.
Website: itunes.apple.com/us/app/ieatout-gluten-free-allergy-free/id323390509?mt=8

Substitutions
This app is only available on the App Store for iOS devices for baking or cooking food, making drinks, and food shopping or dining.
Website: itunes.apple.com/us/app/substitutions/id372387251?mt=8

Yummly Recipes
This app matches over 1 million recipes to your cooking lifestyle's nutrition, diet, food allergies, and favorite cuisines. With Yummly, create a personal food experience that finds the recipes you want, when you want them from thousands of the world's top recipe sites and blogs.
Website: play.google.com/store/apps/details?id=com.yummly.android&hl=en

Index

Index

Page numbers that appear in *Italics* refer to tables or illustrations. Page numbers that have a small 'n' after the page number refer to citation information shown as Notes. Page numbers that appear in **Bold** refer to information contained in boxes within the chapters.

A

AAFA *see* Asthma and Allergy Foundation of America

AAIA *see* Allergy and Asthma Information Association

AANMA *see* Allergy and Asthma Network Mothers of Asthmatics

Academy of Nutrition and Dietetics, contact 329

Accolate (zafirlukast), leukotriene receptor antagonists 55

acupuncture, allergic rhinitis 73

acute urticaria *see* urticaria

age factor
 calcium intake by age group *162*
 food allergy among U.S. children **5**
 nickel health effects **232**
 pet or pest allergens **200**

Agency for Healthcare Research and Quality (AHRQ), contact 325

airways
 asthma **81**
 chronic cough **64**
 cough 63
 described 17
 epinephrine injections 57
 hypersensitivity pneumonitis 91

airways, *continued*
 respiratory system 17
 seasonal allergies 261

alcohol
 allergen patch test 38
 atopic dermatitis 113
 lanolin 245
 sulfite sensitivity 189

alcoholic beverages
 food labelling 130
 sulfite sensitivity 189

allergen immunotherapy *see* allergy shots

allergen patch tests, overview 37–40

"Allergenics—Allergen Patch Tests" (FDA) 37n

allergens
 allergen patch test 37
 allergist 29
 allergy blood test 41
 allergy shots and children 47
 allergy shots/drops 48
 asthma and allergies 81
 breathing problem 255
 climate change and respiratory allergies 123
 cockroach allergy 209
 coughing 63
 dietitian 313
 dust mite allergy 214

allergens, *continued*
    epinephrine injections 57
    FALCPA 299
    food allergens list 127
    food diary 317
    immunotherapy **54**
    indoor air quality 263
    lanolin allergy 245
    pets and asthma 199
    pink eye 97
    seasonal allergies 259
    sulfite sensitivity 187
    vernal keratoconjunctivitis **100**
Allergic Living Magazine, contact 329
allergic reactions
    allergic rhinitis 75
    allergist 27
    allergy and immune system 3
    atopic dermatitis **112**
    cosmetics safety 274
    egg allergy 168
    epinephrine injections 57
    food allergies 127
    fragrance allergies 243
    hair dye allergy 236
    hives 116
    indoor air quality 265
    peanut and tree nut allergies 138
    seafood allergy 156
    seasonal allergies 259
    sting allergies 221
    sulfite sensitivity 187
allergic rhinitis
    allergic reactions 27
    allergy shots 45
    breathing problems 256
    dust mites 214
    leukotriene receptor antagonists 55
    overview 71–5
    sneezing and allergy **66**
    soy allergy 146
AllergicChild.com, contact 329
allergies
    allergy shots 45
    blood test 41
    causes 255
    defined 14
    food allergy 127
    food diary 317
    medications for allergic symptoms 53

allergies, *continued*
    overview 3–5
    patch tests 37
"Allergies" (CDC) 3n
"Allergies" (FDA) 71n
allergist, overview 27–9
allergy *see* allergies
"Allergy" (NIH) 3n
Allergy and Asthma Information Association
    (AAIA), contact 330
Allergy and Asthma Network Mothers of Asthmatics
    (AANMA), contact 330
Allergy Basket, mobile app 339
allergy blood test, overview 41–3
"Allergy Blood Test" (NIH) 41n
allergy drops
    immunotherapy 48
    tabulated *49*
allergy injection, allergy prevention 4
Allergy Reality: Food Safety, mobile app 339
allergy shots
    breathing problems 257
    dust mite allergy 214
    overview 45–52
    sting allergies 225
    see also immunotherapy
"Allergy Shots And Allergy Drops For Adults And
    Children" (HHS) 45n
Allergy UK, contact 330
alveoli
    hypersensitivity pneumonitis 87
    lungs and blood vessels 19
American Academy of Allergy, Asthma and
    Immunology (AAAAI), contact 330
American Academy of Dermatology (AAD),
    contact 331
American Academy of Otolaryngology-Head and
    Neck Surgery (AAO-HNS), contact 331
American Board of Allergy and Immunology (ABAI),
    contact 331
American College of Allergy, Asthma and
    Immunology (ACAAI), contact 331
American Lung Association, contact 332
American Osteopathic College of Dermatology
    (AOCD), contact 332
American Partnership for Eosinophilic Disorders
    (APFED), contact 332
American Rhinologic Society (ARS),
    contact 332

anaphylactic shock
    allergy blood test 41
    food allergies 129
anaphylaxis
    allergic reaction 224
    allergist 28
    allergy 3
    allergy shots 50
    defined **257**
    epinephrine injections 57
    food allergy 128
    latex allergy 104
    overview 119–21
    soy allergy 146
"Anaphylaxis" (NIAID) 119n
antibodies
    adaptive immunity 11
    allergic rhinitis 72
    allergist 27
    allergy blood test 41
    egg allergy 167
    food allergy and related disorders 134
    gluten intolerance 176
    hypersensitivity pneumonitis 86
    seafood allergies 155
    wheat allergy 143
antigens, immune system 11
antihistamines
    allergy attacks **4**
    allergy medicines 53
    allergy shots 47
    atopic dermatitis 112
    breathing problems 257
    egg allergy 169
    lanolin allergy 247
    seasonal allergies 259
    sting allergies 224
    sulfite sensitivity 189
    tabulated *25*
    vernal keratoconjunctivitis 101
arterial blood gas tests, lung function tests 31
Aspergillus, molds 203
aspirin, tabulated *25*
asthma
    allergic reactions 27
    allergy 3
    allergy shots 51
    asthma and allergies 81
    asthma management at school 269

asthma, *continued*
    cockroach allergy 209
    coughing and sneezing 64
    epinephrine injections 59
    immune system reaction 46
    latex allergy 104
    leukotriene receptor antagonists 55
    medications for allergic symptoms 53
    pet allergies 199
    sulfite sensitivity 187
    tabulated *25, 49*
    wheat allergy 143
Asthma and Allergy Foundation of America (AAFA),
    contact 332
"Asthma, Respiratory Allergies and Airway Diseases"
    (NIEHS) 123n
asthma triggers
    asthma and allergies 82
    controlling common asthma triggers in
    schools *271*
    indoor pollutants 267
"Asthma Triggers: Gain Control" (EPA) 199n
atopic dermatitis
    overview 109–14
    skin care at home 291
    see also eczema
"Atopic Dermatitis" (NIAMS) 109n, 287n
autoimmune diseases, defined 14
autoinjectors *see* epinephrine
ayurvedic medicine, allergic rhinitis 74

B

B cells (B lymphocytes)
    immune system 8
    immune system disorders 14
bacteria
    allergic rhinitis 74
    allergy blood test 41
    celiac disease 173
    coughing and sneezing 67
    gluten-free diet **179**
    hypersensitivity pneumonitis 85
    immune system 7
    indoor air quality 263
    pink eye 97
    raw milk and lactose intolerance 166
    seasonal allergies 259
    sinusitis 78

bacteria, *continued*
  sting allergies 221
  urticaria 116
"Bad Bug Book—Handbook Of Foodborne
  Pathogenic Microorganisms And Natural Toxins"
  (FDA) 183n
basophils, immune system 9
BBC Gluten-Free Recipes, website address 337
BBC Nut-Free Recipes, website address 337
BBC Special Diets Recipes, website address 337
"Beware Of Bug Bites And Stings" (FDA) 221n
biological allergens, indoor air quality 263
biopsy
  celiac disease 175
  lymphangioleiomyomatosis (LAM) 34
bird fancier's lung *see* hypersensitivity pneumonitis
blood gas tests, lung function tests 31
blood pressure
  allergy shots/drops **48**
  anaphylaxis **119**
  cough 65
  epinephrine injections 57
  food allergies 129, **293**
  immune system 15
  seafood allergy 156
  soy allergy 145
blood tests
  allergic rhinitis 72
  allergist 29
  allergy blood test 41
  celiac disease 175
  food allergy **293**
  gluten intolerance 176
  hypersensitivity pneumonitis 90
  lymphangioleiomyomatosis (LAM) 34
blood vessels
  anaphylaxis **119**
  epinephrine injections 57
  hypersensitivity pneumonitis 87
  pink eye 97
  respiratory system 17
blurred vision, eye allergies 99
breastfeeding
  breathing problems 256
  epinephrine injections 59
breathing
  described 20
  epinephrine injections 60
  lung function tests 31
  respiratory system 17

breathing muscles, described 19
bronchi, respiratory system 18
bronchial tubes
  asthma and school attendance **269**
  respiratory system 18
bronchiectasis, described **64**
bronchioles, lungs and blood vessels 19
bronchoalveolar lavage, hypersensitivity
  pneumonitis 90
bronchodilators
  cough medicines **69**
  egg allergy 169
  hypersensitivity pneumonitis 93

C

calcium, lactose intolerance 165
"Calcium" (NIH) 159n
Canadian Lung Association, contact 333
CDC *see* Centers for Disease Control and Prevention
celiac disease, overview 171–81
Celiac Disease Foundation, contact 333
cells, immune system 7
Center for Food Safety and Applied Nutrition
  (CFSAN), contact 325
Centers for Disease Control and Prevention (CDC)
  contact 326
  publications
    allergies 3n
    asthma management in schools 269n
    contact dermatitis and latex allergy 103n
    egg allergies and vaccines 319n
    formaldehyde allergy 249n
    going out to eat with food allergies 305n
    mold 203n
    nickel allergy 227n
    pink eye 97n
    sinusitis 77n
challenge test, described 29
chronic bronchitis, chronic cough **64**
chronic obstructive pulmonary disease (COPD),
  chronic cough **64**
cigarette smoke, irritants 65
"Cigarette Smoke" (NIEHS) 217n
climate change, respiratory allergies 123
clothing, formaldehyde allergy 251
cockroach allergy, overview 209–12
"Cockroaches" (NIEHS) 209n
cold *see* common cold

"Cold, Flu, Or Allergy?" (NIH) 23n
color additives, described 278
common cold
    acute cough 67
    sinus infection 78
computed axial tomography scan (CAT scan; CT scan), hypersensitivity pneumonitis 90
condoms, latex allergies 5
congestion, allergic rhinitis **71**
conjunctivitis (pink eye), described 97
"Consumer Updates—What FDA Learned About Dark Chocolate And Milk Allergies" (FDA) 149n
contact dermatitis, overview 103–7
contact lens, eye allergy 99
contaminated foods, hypersensitivity pneumonitis 86
Cook IT Allergy Free, website address 337
COPD *see* chronic obstructive pulmonary disease
Corn-Free Recipes, website address 337
corticosteroids
    atopic dermatitis 290
    eosinophilic esophagitis 134
    hypersensitivity pneumonitis 93
    sulfite sensitivity 189
    urticaria **116**
    see also nasal corticosteroids
cosmetics
    gluten intolerance 178
    safety 273
"Cosmetics—Hair Dyes" (FDA) 235n
"Cosmetics—Nail Care Products" (FDA) 283n
"Cosmetics—Novelty Makeup" (FDA) 277n
"Cosmetics—Using Cosmetics Safely" (FDA) 273n
"Cough" (NHLBI) 63n
cough suppressants **69**
coughing
    allergic rhinitis 71
    anaphylaxis 120
    food allergies 129
    hay fever 72
    latex allergy 104
    overview 63–70
    seafood allergies 156
    sinusitis 77
    smoke irritation 217
    sulfite sensitivity 188
    treatment 67
"Cracking the Peanut Allergy—USDA Program Provides Doctors A Way To Help Children" (USDA) 137n

cromolyn sodium
    respiratory allergy 259
    vernal keratoconjunctivitis 101
cross contact, food allergies 131
crusting, pink eye 98
cytokines
    cancer 15
    immune tolerance 13
    sepsis 15

D

dairy-free products
    food labels 151
    online recipe resources 337
    see also milk allergy
Dairy Free Cakes, website address 337
Dairy-Free Dinner Recipes, website address 337
Dairy-Free Recipes, website address 338
dander
    pet allergies 199
    trigger control **270**
dark chocolate allergy, described 149
decongestants
    described 54
    respiratory allergy treatment 259
dendritic cells, innate immunity 11
dermatitis herpetiformis, described 174
diaphragm, breathing 19
diarrhea
    allergic reactions 28
    blood test 42
    exercise-induced anaphylaxis 120
    wheat allergy 143
diet
    atopic dermatitis 113
    celiac disease treatment 177
    eosinophilic esophagitis 134
    gluten intolerance 177
    lactose intolerance 165
    peanut and tree nut allergies 139
    soy allergy 146
    wheat allergy 143
    working with a dietitian 313
dietary supplements
    calcium 165
    soy 145
dietitians, overview 313–5

dining out
    celiac disease 180
    egg allergy 168
    The Food Allergen Labeling And Consumer Protection Act (FALCPA) 303
    peanut allergies 139
    seafood allergy 156
"Digestive Diseases—Celiac Disease" (NIDDK) 171n
drug overlap, flu 24
"Drug Record—Leukotriene Receptor Antagonists" (NIH) 53n
dust mite allergy, overview 213–5
"Dust Mites" (NIEHS) 213n

E

Eating With Food Allergies, website address 338
eczema
    overview 109–14
    skin care concerns 287
    wet wrap therapy 291
    see also atopic dermatitis
"Eczema—Eczema" (Atopic Dermatitis) Treatment" (NIAID) 287n
egg allergy
    overview 167–9
    vaccine recommendations 320
"Egg Allergy" (Omnigraphics) 167n
Egg-Free Recipes, website address 338
elimination diet, food allergy **293**
emergency care, life-threatening anaphylactic reactions 168
eosinophilic esophagitis, described 134
eosinophils, innate immune cells 11
EPA *see* U.S. Environmental Protection Agency
epiglottis, function 18
epinephrine
    anaphylaxis 51, 116
    emergency medication 29
    exercise-induced anaphylaxis (EIAn) 120
    injection overdose symptoms 60
    overview 57–60
    peanut allergy 138
"Epinephrine Injections For Life-Threatening Allergic Reactions" (Omnigraphics) 57n
essential oils, described 242
exercise
    asthma 261

exercise, *continued*
    hive 116
    hypersensitivity pneumonitis 95
exercise-induced anaphylaxis (EIAn), described 120
"Exercise-Induced Anaphylaxis" (NCATS) 119n
exhalation, described 20
expectorants, cough medicines **69**
expiration date, cosmetic labels 274
eye allergies, overview 97–101
eye cosmetics, safety concerns **274**

F

face paints, overview 277–82
fatigue
    flu 23
    hypersensitivity pneumonitis 94
    sinus infection 77
    vibratory urticaria **116**
FDA *see* U.S. Food and Drug Administration
"FDA Approves Odactra For House Dust Mite Allergies" (FDA) 213n
fire ants, insect sting allergies 5
flu, overview 23–5
flush, anaphylaxis 5
food additives, allergen labeling requirements 301
Food Allergen Labeling and Consumer Protection Act (FALCPA)
    food allergens 300
    overview 299–303
    soy **146**
"Food Allergen Labeling And Consumer Protection Act Of 2004 Questions And Answers" (FDA) 299n
food allergy
    eosinophilic esophagitis 134
    food allergy among U.S. children **5**
    food allergy and related disorders 133
    immune tolerance 12
    overview 127–31
    see also oral allergy syndrome
Food Allergy and Intolerance Self-Diagnosis, website address 338
Food Allergy Canada, contact 333
"Food Allergy—Characterizing Food Allergy And Addressing Related Disorders" (NIAID) 133n
food allergy lab, overview 309–11
"Food Allergy Lab Fits On Your Keychain" (NIBIB) 309n
Food Allergy Kitchen, website address 338

Food Allergy Research & Education® (FARE), contact 333

Food Allergy Research & Education® (FARE): Life With Food Allergies, website address 338

Food Allergy Research and Resource Program (FARRP), contact 334

"Food And Drug Administration Department Of Health And Human Services Subchapter C—Drugs: General" (FDA) 187n

food diary, overview 317–8

"A Food Diary Can Reduce Risk Of Reactions" (Omnigraphics) 317n

"Food—Food Allergies: What You Need To Know" (FDA) 127n

food intolerance
lactose 159
versus food allergy 135

food labels
food allergies 139
gluten-free diet 180
law 128
soy allergy 146

food poisoning, described 134

"For Consumers—Allergy Relief For Your Child" (FDA) 45n

"For Consumers—FDA: Foods Must Contain What Label Says" (FDA) 293n

"For Consumers—Have Food Allergies? Read the Label" (FDA) 293n

"For Consumers—Problems Digesting Dairy Products?" (FDA) 159n

"For Consumers—Seasonal Allergies: Which Medication Is Right For You?" (FDA) 53n

"For Consumers—Think Before You Ink: Are Tattoos Safe?" (FDA) 277n

formaldehyde allergy, overview 249–52

fragrance allergy, overview 241–3

"Fragrances In Cosmetics" (FDA) 241n

"Frequently Asked Questions—Contact Dermatitis And Latex Allergy" (CDC) 103n

fungi
disease-causing organisms 27
hypersensitivity pneumonitis 85
molds 203

G

gastroesophageal reflux disease (GERD), chronic cough 64

gelatin, sulfite sensitivity 189

genetic immune disorders, immune-compromised people 8

gloves
contact dermatitis 103
latex allergies 5

Gluten-Free Cake Recipes, website address 338

gluten-free diet, described 177

Gluten Free Food Finder, mobile app 339

Gluten-Free Lunch Recipes, website address 338

Gluten-Free Snack Recipes, website address 338

gluten intolerance, overview 171–80

"Going Out to Eat with Food Allergies" (CDC) 305n

grass pollen, described 196

H

hair dye allergy, overview 235–9

hay fever *see* allergic rhinitis

headache, drug overlap 24

"Health Topics—Pulmonary Function Tests" (NHLBI) 31n

Healthfinder®, contact 326

"Healthy Schools—Asthma In Schools" (CDC) 269n

heartburn, eosinophilic esophagitis 134

henna, color additives 238

histamine
described 53
food allergy 317
hives 116

histamine poisoning, overview 183–5

hives, overview 115–7

HLA *see* human leukocyte antigens

"How The Lungs Work" (NHLBI) 17n

"How To Control Your Seasonal Allergies" (NIH) 259n

"How To Safely Use Nail Care Products" (FDA) 283n

human leukocyte antigens (HLA), immune tolerance 13

humidity, molds 204

hypersensitivity pneumonitis, overview 85–96

"Hypersensitivity Pneumonitis" (NHLBI) 85n

hypersensitivity reactions, described 14

I

iEatOut Gluten Free & Allergy Free, mobile app 339

immune memory 10

immune response
    allergen immunotherapy 55
    diagnostic tests 91
    genetics 88
    seasonal allergies 261
immune system
    allergic rhinitis 71
    allergic symptom treatment 53
    allergies 7–17
    allergy blood tests 41
    atopic dermatitis 290
    egg allergy 167
    food allergy 135
    hives 116
    hypersensitivity pneumonitis 85
    lung transplants 94
    nickel 232
    seafood allergies 155
    vernal keratoconjunctivitis 101
"Immune System Research" (NIAID) 7n
immunoglobulin E (IgE) antibodies
    allergic reactions 29
    allergy blood tests 41
    food allergies 134
    seasonal allergies 259
    soy allergy 145
immunotherapy
    overview 45–52
    seasonal allergies 259
indoor air quality, management 263
"Indoor Air Quality (IAQ)—Biological Pollutants'
    Impact On Indoor Air Quality" (EPA) 263n
inflammation
    hypersensitivity pneumonitis 85
    innate immunity 11
    pink eye 97
    seasonal allergies 261
    sulfite sensitivity 187
    wheat allergy 143
inhalation
    nickel 230
    sulfite sensitivity 188
insect repellent 223
insect stings, allergy 3
integrated exogenous antigen testing (iEAT), food
    allergies 310
intercostal muscles, breathing 19
International Food Information Council (IFIC),
    contact 334

irritants
    atopic dermatitis 111
    cough 63
    pink eye 98
    sinus infections 78
    skin care 291
    smoking 217
"Is It Food Allergy Or Food Intolerance?" (VA) 133n
itching
    allergic contact dermatitis 106
    allergic rhinitis 71
    allergy shots 50
    hives 116
    insect bites 224
    oral allergy syndrome 133
    scombrotoxin **184**

J

jewelry, nickel allergy 227
joint pain
    hypersensitivity pneumonitis 89
    sulfite sensitivity 188

K

Kids With Food Allergies
    contact 334
    website address 338

L

lactose intolerance
    celiac disease 175
    overview 159–66
"LAM—Diagnosis" (NHLBI) 31n
lanolin allergy, overview 245–7
"Lanolin Allergy" (Omnigraphics) 245n
latex allergy, overview 103–7
lecithin, soy allergy 147
leukotriene receptor antagonists (LTRAs),
    described 55
levocabastine, vernal keratoconjunctivitis 101
lifestyle changes
    anaphylaxis 121
    cough 68
    follow-up care 94

light therapy
    atopic dermatitis **112**
    skin care 290
lightheadedness
    epinephrine 320
    food allergies 129
    seafood allergies 156
Living Without, website address 338
Livostin (levocabastine), vernal
  keratoconjunctivitis 101
lung diffusion capacity, defined 31
lung function tests
    hypersensitivity pneumonitis 91
    overview 31–5
lung irritants, respiratory control center 21
lungs
    asthma **81**
    climate change 123
    hypersensitivity pneumonitis 86
    immune system reaction 46
    molds 204
    nickel 229
    pulmonary function tests 31
    respiratory system 17
Lyme disease, sting allergies 221
lymph nodes
    lung function tests 35
    lymphatic system 10
lymphatic system, immune system 10
lymphocytes
    bone marrow 9
    cancer 15
lymphoid organ, lymphatic system 10

M

macrophages
    immune system 9
    leukotriene receptor antagonists 55
major histocompatibility complex (MHC), immune
  tolerance 13
makeup
    atopic dermatitis 113
    cosmetics 273
    face painting 277
    lanolin allergy **246**
    pink eye 99
"Managing Asthma In The School Environment"
  (EPA) 269n

"Managing Pests In Schools—Cockroaches And
  Schools" (EPA) 209n
mast cells
    anaphylaxis **119**
    cysteinyl leukotrienes 55
    immune system 11
medical history
    atopic dermatitis 111
    egg allergy 319
    hypersensitivity pneumonitis 90
    lactose intolerance 164
    latex allergy *105*
    skin care 288
    sulfite sensitivity 188
medications
    allergic reactions 28
    allergic rhinitis 75
    asthma 269
    atopic dermatitis **112**
    contact dermatitis 106
    dust mites 214
    epinephrine injections 59
    food allergies 318
    nail care 285
    sulfite sensitivity 187
MHC *see* major histocompatibility complex
milk allergy
    food allergies 167
    lactose intolerance **159**
moisture control, indoor air quality 265
moisturizers
    lanolin allergy **246**
    skin care 291
"Mold—Basic Facts" (CDC) 203n
monocytes, immune system 11
monosodium glutamate (MSG), wheat allergy 144
multiple sinus infections *see* sinusitis

N

nail care, cosmetic product safety 283
nail curing lamps, described 284
nasal corticosteroids
    allergy attacks 54
    see also corticosteroids
nasal growths, chronic sinusitis 79
nasal pruritus, allergic rhinitis 71
nasal spray, pollen allergies **196**
nasal spray flu vaccine, egg allergy **322**

nasal steroids, airborne allergy 25
National Center for Advancing Translational Sciences (NCATS)
    publications
        exercise-induced anaphylaxis 119n
        vernal keratoconjunctivitis 97n
National Center for Complementary and Integrative Health (NCCIH)
    contact 326
    publication
        seasonal allergies 71n
National Center for Environmental Health (NCEH), contact 326
National Digestive Diseases Information Clearinghouse (NDDIC), contact 326
National Eczema Association (NEA), contact 334
National Heart, Lung, and Blood Institute (NHLBI)
    contact 327
    publications
        cough 63n
        hypersensitivity pneumonitis 85n
        lung function tests 31n
        pulmonary function tests 31n
        respiratory system 17n
National Institute of Allergy and Infectious Diseases (NIAID)
    contact 327
    publications
        anaphylaxis 119n
        eczema (atopic dermatitis) treatment 287n
        food allergy and related disorders 133n
        immune system 7n
National Institute of Arthritis and Musculoskeletal and Skin Diseases (NIAMS)
    contact 327
    publications
        atopic dermatitis 109n, 287n
National Institute of Biomedical Imaging and Bioengineering (NIBIB)
    publication
        food allergy lab fits on your keychain 309n
National Institute of Diabetes and Digestive and Kidney Disorders (NIDDK)
    contact 327
    publication
        celiac disease 171n

National Institute of Environmental Health Sciences (NIEHS)
    contact 328
    publications
        cigarette smoke 217n
        climate change and respiratory allergies 123n
        cockroaches 209n
        dust mites 213n
        pets and animals 199n
        pollen 195n
National Institutes of Health (NIH)
    contact 328
    publications
        allergy 3n
        allergy blood test 41n
        breathing problems 255n
        calcium 159n
        cold, flu, or allergy 23n
        contact dermatitis 103n
        leukotriene receptor antagonists 53n
        seasonal allergies 259n
National Jewish Medical and Research Center, contact 334
natural killer cells (NK cells)
    defined 9
    immune deficiencies 14
NHLBI *see* National Heart, Lung, and Blood Institute
NIAID *see* National Institute of Allergy and Infectious Diseases
NIAMS *see* National Institute of Arthritis and Musculoskeletal and Skin Diseases
nickel allergy
    children 232
    overview 227–33
NK cells *see* natural killer cells
novelty makeup, safety concerns 277

O

Office of Disease Prevention and Health Promotion (ODPHP)
    publication
        asthma and allergies 81n
Omnigraphics
    publications
        egg allergy 167n
        epinephrine injections 57n

Omnigraphics
    publications, *continued*
        food diary 317n
        lanolin allergy 245n
        peanut and tree nut allergies 137n
        sulfite sensitivity 187n
        urticaria (hives) 115n
        visiting an allergist 27n
        working with a dietitian 313n
opioids, hypersensitivity pneumonitis 93
oral allergy syndrome, described 133
oral food challenge, food intolerance 139

P

Pan American Allergy Society (PAAS), contact 335
Pan American Health Organization, contact 335
papules, patch tests 39
patch tests
    contact dermatitis *105*
    hair dye allergy 238
    lanolin allergy 246
    overview 37–40
peanut allergy
    immunotherapy **50**
    overview 137–41
"Peanut And Tree Nut Allergies"
    (Omnigraphics) 137n
Peanut Free Recipes, website address 338
PeanutAllergy.com, contact 335
perfumes
    atopic dermatitis 113
    cough 63
    eczema 288
    sting allergies 222
pests
    asthma 83
    asthma triggers in schools *271*
    pet allergy **200**
pet allergy, overview 199–201
pet dander
    eye allergies 97
    food diary 318
"Pets And Animals" (NIEHS) 199n
phthalates, fragrance allergies 243
physical examination
    seafood allergies 156
    sinusitis 79
    sulfite sensitivity 188

pink eye *see* conjunctivitis
"Pink Eye: Usually Mild And Easy To Treat" (CDC) 97n
pneumonia, chest X-ray 67
pollen, allergic rhinitis 71
"Pollen" (NIEHS) 195n
pollen allergies
    allergy shots 46
    complementary health approaches 73
    overview 195–8
pollen counts, allergy medicines 53
Pollen.com, contact 335
polyps, sinusitis 78
postnasal drip
    defined 64
    sinusitis 77
precipitin test, hypersensitivity pneumonitis 91
pregnancy, epinephrine 59
"Prevent Allergies And Asthma Attacks At Home"
    (ODPHP) 81n
processed/prepackaged food
    egg allergy 168
    food diary 318
    gluten intolerance 171
    soy allergy 145
pseudoephedrine, allergy medicines 54
psoriasis, contact dermatitis 106
pulmonary fibrosis, hypersensitivity pneumonitis 88
pulmonary function test (PFT), overview 31–5
pulmonary hypertension, hypersensitivity
    pneumonitis 90
pulse oximetry
    defined 32
    lymphangioleiomyomatosis 33

R

ragweed
    allergy preventive strategies 195
    oral allergy syndrome 133
raw milk, lactose intolerance **166**
rebound effect, nasal decongestants 54
recipes
    eating out with allergies 306
    online resources 337
"Red, Itchy Rash?" (NIH) 103n
remissions, atopic dermatitis 109
respiratory system
    depicted *18*
    overview 17–21

restaurant *see* dining out
rhinitis
    allergy shots 45
    sneezing **66**
risk factors
    allergic rhinitis 74
    hypersensitivity pneumonitis 87
    sinus 78
    wheat allergy 144
runny/stuffy nose, allergy blood test 42

S

safety concerns, hair dye allergy **235**
scaling, atopic dermatitis 287
scented soaps, sting allergies 222
schools, asthma management 269
seafood allergy, overview 155–7
"Seafood Allergy" (Omnigraphics) 155n
seasonal allergic rhinitis, described 45
seasonal allergies
    allergic rhinitis 71
    allergy medicines 53
    control 259
    defined 53
"Seasonal Allergies At A Glance" (NCCIH) 71n
secondhand smoke, irritants 63
"Seeking Allergy Relief" (NIH) 255n
seizures, anaphylaxis **257**
sepsis, described 15
shellfish, food allergens 128
shock, anaphylaxis **257**
shortness of breath, asthma 261
side effects
    allergic rhinitis 74
    allergy shots 50
    epinephrine 59
    nasal corticosteroids 54
"Sinus Infection" (Sinusitis)" (CDC) 77n
sinusitis, overview 77–9
skin care
    atopic dermatitis 112
    eczema 287
    see also contact dermatitis
skin prick test
    egg allergy 168
    seafood allergies 156
    soy allergy 146

skin tests
    allergic rhinitis 72
    peanut and tree nut allergies 139
    sulfite sensitivity 188
sneezing
    allergy blood test 41
    allergy shots 45
    dust mite allergy 214
    seasonal allergies **259**
    soy allergy 146
    sulfite sensitivity 188
soaps and detergents, atopic dermatitis 111
socks/shoes, sting allergies 222
sore throat, formaldehyde allergy **250**
soy allergy, overview 145–7
"Soy Allergy" (Omnigraphics) 145n
spirometry
    depicted *32*
    described 31
spleen
    defined 10
    celiac disease 174
spores
    asthma 271
    described 203
    seasonal allergies 259
sting allergy, overview 221–5
stress, eczema 288
sublingual therapy, allergy medicines 55
Substitutions, mobile app 339
Sudafed (pseudoephedrine), allergy medicines 54
sulfite sensitivity, overview 187–91
"Sulfite Sensitivity" (Omnigraphics) 187n
sulfites
    food 189
    epinephrine injections 59
    sulfite sensitivity 188
sun exposure
    food diary 318
    urticaria **116**
sun protection factor (SPF), curing lamps 285

T

T cells (T lymphocytes)
    defined 9
    egg allergy 167
    immune deficiencies 13

tattoos
  color additives 238
  ghoulish glow 279
  safety concerns 280
temporary tattoos, safety concerns 238
tests
  allergic rhinitis 72
  allergies 72
  arterial blood gas tests 32
  celiac disease 175
  cough 67
  egg allergy 168
  hypersensitivity pneumonitis 91
  lactose intolerance 164
  lung function 31
  lymphangioleiomyomatosis 33
  patch test 37
  peanut and tree nut allergies 139
thickened skin, contact dermatitis *105*
tingling, food allergies 129
toll-like receptors, described 10
topical corticosteroids *see* corticosteroids
toxic chemicals, irritant contact dermatitis *104*
"Toxic Substances Portal—Formaldehyde—ToxFAQs"
  (CDC) 249n
"Toxic Substances Portal—Nickel" (CDC) 227n
tree nut allergy, overview 137–9
tree pollen, described 197
triggers
  allergies 256
  asthma 269
  celiac disease **177**
  urticaria **116**
T.R.U.E. test, described 37
20 Tried-and-True Egg-Free Desserts, website
  address 338

U

ultraviolet rays (UV rays)
  nail care 284
  T.R.U.E. test 38
upper airway cough syndrome (UACS)
  chronic cough 68
  medical conditions 64
urticaria (hives)
  allergy blood test 42
  egg allergy 167

urticaria (hives), *continued*
  epinephrine injections 57
  exercise-induced anaphylaxis 120
  food allergies 129
  latex allergy 104
  overview 115–7
  peanut allergy 137
  scombrotoxin 184
  sulfite sensitivity 188
"Urticaria (Hives)" (Omnigraphics) 115n
U.S. Department of Agriculture (USDA)
  contact 328
  publication
    peanut and tree nut allergies 137n
U.S. Department of Health and Human Services
  (HHS)
  publications
    allergy shots 45n
    immune system 7n
U.S. Department of Veterans Affairs (VA)
  publication
    food allergy or food intolerance 133n
U.S. Environmental Protection Agency (EPA)
  contact 328
  publications
    cockroach allergy 209n
    indoor air quality 263n
    managing asthma in schools 269n
    pet allergies 199n
U.S. Food and Drug Administration (FDA)
  contact 328
  publications
    allergen patch tests 37n
    allergies 71n
    allergy shots 45n
    bug bites and stings 221n
    cosmetics safety 273n
    dark chocolate and milk allergies 149n
    dust mites 213n
    face painting and tattoos 277n
    The Food Allergen Labeling and Consumer
      Protection Act (FALCPA) 299n
    food allergies 127n
    food label 293n
    fragrance allergy 241n
    hair dyes 235n
    lactose intolerance 159n
    nail care products 283n
    scombrotoxin (histamine) poisoning 183n

U.S. Food and Drug Administration (FDA)
publications, *continued*
seasonal allergy medication 53n
sulfite sensitivity 187n
U.S. National Library of Medicine (NLM),
contact 329

V

vaccination
atopic dermatitis 113
described 12
egg allergy 321
smallpox 290
ventilation systems
indoor air quality 265
hypersensitivity pneumonitis 86
vernal keratoconjunctivitis (VKC), described **100**
"Vernal Keratoconjunctivitis" (NCATS) 97n
Vickerstaff Health Services, contact 335
villi, gluten-free diet 177
vitamin D, lactose intolerance **165**
vomiting
allergy blood test 42
anaphylaxis 120
egg allergy 168
epinephrine injection 59
food allergies 129
peanut allergy 138
scombrotoxin 184
seafood allergy 156
soy allergy 146

W

"What Is The Immune System?" (HHS) 7n
wheat allergy
celiac disease **171**
overview 143–4
"Wheat Allergy?" (Omnigraphics) 143n

Wheat-Free Recipes, website address 338
wheezing
allergy blood test 42
allergy shots 50
anaphylaxis 120
egg allergy 167
epinephrine injections 57
hay fever *73*
latex allergy 104
seafood allergy 156
seasonal allergies 261
soy allergy 146
sulfite sensitivity 188
"When You Should See An Allergist"
(Omnigraphics) 27n
wool alcohol, lanolin allergy 246
wool or synthetic fibers
atopic dermatitis 111
dust mites 213
lanolin allergy 245
skin care 291
"Working With A Dietitian" (Omnigraphics) 313n
World Allergy Organization (WAO), contact 335

X

X-linked severe combined immunodeficiency (SCID),
immune system 14
X-ray
gastroesophageal reflux disease (GERD) 67
hypersensitivity pneumonitis 91

Y

Yummly Recipes, mobile app 339

Z

zafirlukast, leukotriene receptor antagonists 55